THE TREE OF SYMPTOMS

Dr. Emil Šabanović

Preface

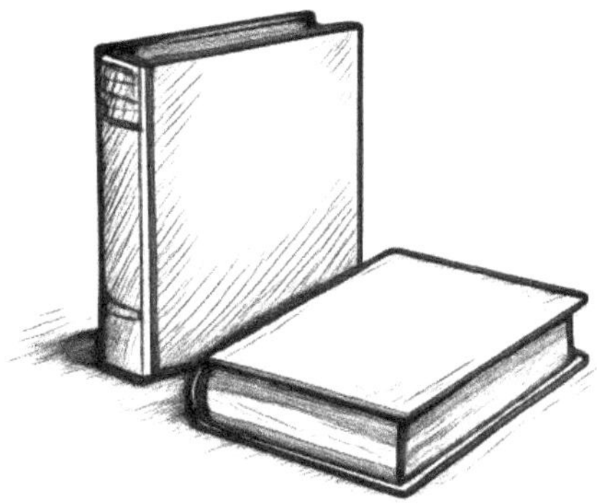

Remember how it felt, as a child, to be curious about the world? You watched a caterpillar turn into a butterfly and wanted to know *how.* You wondered why a bee dies after stinging, or why rain smells the way it does. That curiosity was pure, untouched by pressure or purpose.

Now imagine you never lost it. You studied medicine or psychology, carried that same curiosity into the study of human beings. You learned how systems connect, how bodies and minds adapt. You kept going, step by step, until you reached your highest level: a professor in the university hospital, leading research and teaching others what you've discovered. You felt fulfilled, proud to finally understand so much about how a person works, and eager to share it. Then one day, under your latest publication, a patient reads the title and types a single word: *Bullshit.* And you realize how far our language has drifted. We built towers of knowledge so high that patients can no longer find the entrance. Even colleagues working directly with patients struggle to translate. Some patients end up trusting health workers who don't understand themselves. When a patient tells me, *"After twenty years of therapy, finally someone explained it,"* I feel a quiet obligation. If I can make complex things clear without flattening them, maybe that is my actual work. That is why I write, to give colleagues ways to speak to patients without losing accuracy or warmth. And if this text stirred something in you, imagine what happens when a patient hears a comparison crafted for their own story. Suddenly psychoeducation stops being a theory. It becomes something human, alive and authentic.

This book grew out of my everyday work with patients; conversations that often began with symptoms the body could no longer hide. Fatigue, pain, dizziness, palpitations, stories that circled through endless tests and still had no name. Over time, I realized that what helped most was not one method or diagnosis, but understanding how body, mind and story belong together. The title *The Tree of Symptoms* was not planned. It came from a simple image I created for my patients: a tree showing symptoms in the leaves, development and behavior in the trunk, deeper roots reaching into biology and the soil to represent transgenerational influences. On the table in our waiting room lay printed copies of that drawing. People kept taking them. We printed more and, again, they disappeared. Eventually, I understood why. This picture made sense of something that explanations often could not. It showed how symptoms grow from somewhere and that they can also change. I kept the original tree image with its simple outline for this book, even though I could now take the time to make a more polished version. I chose to stay with the one that worked for patients, the one they kept taking from the waiting room table. It feels more real and it carries the same spirit in which this book was written. That small tree became the seed of this book.

The cases in this book are drawn from real clinical experience, but none describe a single individual in full. They are composites, carefully shaped from fragments of different encounters to illustrate the central idea of each section. This approach protects privacy, especially because some stories in psychosomatic medicine are so distinctive that a person could be recognized. And some patients are publicly known. The aim is not to present personal histories, but to convey the patterns and principles that can help us understand complex symptoms and their meaning. Although I wrote this book alone, I did not write it in isolation. Along the way, I received thoughtful feedback from colleagues across different areas of medicine. Their insights helped shape these pages into something practical, a text that can speak to physicians, psychotherapists, nurses and all who meet patients whose suffering cannot be explained by tests alone.

Approach this book as you would the birth of something not yet fully known. It will not arrive all at once. Some ideas will feel familiar; others may surprise you. When different ways of understanding begin to weave together - medicine, psychotherapy and biology - they no longer remain what they were. Research increasingly supports such integration: rather than strict adherence to a single school, using flexible, evidence-based collaboration leads to better outcomes, especially for patients with complex psychosomatic conditions. The field is moving from purity of method toward coherence of understanding and that is where this book begins. If you are new to the topic, read slowly, as if following signs through unfamiliar terrain. And if you already work with these patients, I hope you will find something here that deepens your practice, a way to see more clearly, to listen more closely, and to remember that even in the most complex cases, healing begins the moment we understand.

I come from Montenegro, where I studied medicine, first learning the foundations of the body, but always drawn to the story behind the symptoms. Later, in Switzerland, I completed my specializations in psychiatry, psychotherapy, psychosomatic and psychosocial medicine. Those years brought scientific discipline together with the everyday realities of practice. Between the two, a new way of seeing began to form, one that this book now tries to share.

This book was never meant to follow the logic of a manual. It moves more like a story, tracing how body and mind speak through one another. The chapters do not march through theory; they wander, return, and connect, as real practice does. You will find science here, but not as a list of citations. The research is built into the language, in the way we explain things to patients and to ourselves. Some images return more than once because they live at the core of psychosomatic work, the same truths seen from different angles. My hope is that this rhythm, clinical, reflective, and at times lyrical, helps the reader not only understand but also *feel* how coherence emerges from complexity. I hope you can enjoy this book and find it useful, no matter what field you work in.

Contents

CHAPTER ONE

Biological Foundations

How To Approach Chapter One

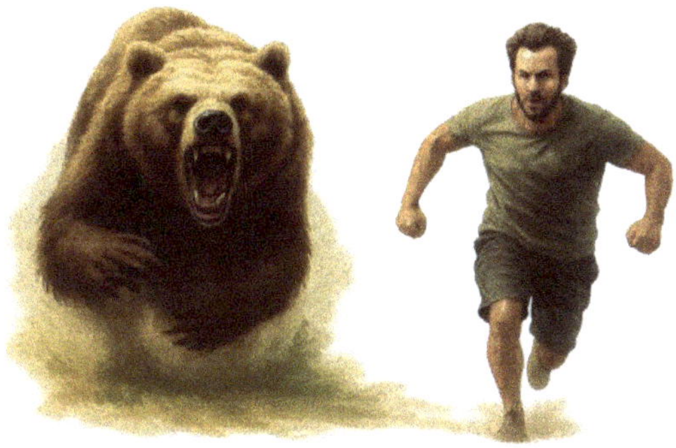

Picture this: you're walking in the forest… the air is calm, the path quiet… Suddenly, out of nowhere, a bear charges toward you. In that instant, survival mode takes over and stress hormones surge through your system. Your autonomic nervous system pushes every cell into high alert. There is no space for emotions; you don't stay there *feeling* fear in that moment. There is also no room for thought; you don't *analyze.* You won't think: *"Wow, this bear is so fast, and it has big claws."* You just run.

When the danger passes, your body begins to settle. First come the physical aftershocks: trembling hands, weak legs, a pounding heart. Then emotions surface: the fear you didn't feel while running, or the relief of having escaped. Finally, the rational mind returns. Now you can reflect: *"that was dangerous; maybe I'll take another path next time."*

But what happens if you're running from a bear for five years? Or ten? Or your whole life? The body and brain adjust to constant threat, until increased alertness becomes the new normal. Feelings grow dull or blocked. Thought narrows into short-term coping and the prefrontal cortex yields to limbic control, leaving little space for creativity, planning, or reflection. A lot of people live like this.

Over time, the body itself starts to reshape around survival. Stress hormones keep circulating, slowly wearing down organs and tissues. The balance between activation and recovery skews toward constant alert. Muscles tighten, sleep shortens, digestion falters. The inner alarm stays on too long, reacting to small signals as if they were danger itself. Even gene expression can shift under this pressure, leaving traces of long stress in our cells. And the same forces that keep us alive can, over years, hasten our aging. Human bonds also write themselves into our physiology. Safe relationships calm the inner alarm and teach the body how to settle. But isolation, conflict, or unsafe homes can keep the system on edge just as surely as a predator would. Early experiences of instability or overwhelming stress don't just influence the mind; they sculpt the body's patterns of protection for years to come.

Yet the same biology that encodes suffering can also encode healing. Safety, connection, and new experiences of regulation give the nervous system the chance to reset. The body can learn balance again.

The path ahead leads through that same forest, this time at a calmer pace.

How the Body Pays the Price: Stress Biology Foundations

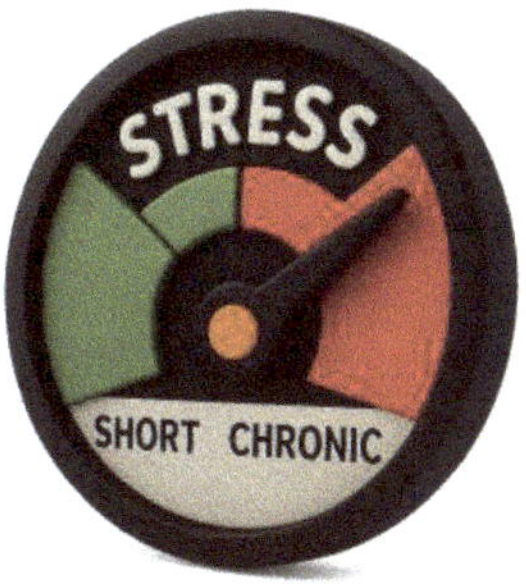

When you face stress, one of the body's key communication lines switches on: the HPA axis, short for hypothalamus, pituitary, and adrenal glands. The hypothalamus senses pressure or threat and signals the pituitary gland. The pituitary passes the message on to the adrenal glands, which release cortisol, the main hormone that sustains endurance. Cortisol mobilizes energy, heightens alertness, and postpones non-essential functions like digestion or reproduction so the body can focus on survival. It helps you care for a sick relative through a long night or stay focused when life demands more than usual.

But when the pressure never ends, the same system begins to turn against you. The HPA axis keeps firing, cortisol stays high, and the body forgets how to switch off. The natural daily rhythm, that's high in the morning and low at night, flattens. The result is a strange mix of exhaustion and inner tension. The immune system weakens, metabolism slows, and sleep no longer restores. Muscles ache, digestion falters, and the mind becomes foggy. Neuroscientist Bruce McEwen called this invisible cost *allostatic load:* the gradual wear and tear that accumulates when the body's stress system never fully resets. Even without dramatic events, daily strain can keep the system running, the constant background noise of obligations, uncertainty, and emotional effort, often amplified by financial or caregiving strain.

For some people, this "always-on" pattern is not new. It can start in childhood. Early experiences of fear, neglect, or chaos teach the body to live in readiness. Years later, the same biological reflex can still govern their physiology, as if the danger never ended. In psychosomatic medicine, this is not a metaphor but a literal imprint: the past continuing to shape the body's present reactions. Cortisol, then, is both guardian and burden. It fuels survival in the short run, but if it never stops flowing, it slowly burns the system from within. How we perceive and interpret stress also shapes this loop.

Case: Anna, The Exhausted Teacher

Anna is 38, a dedicated teacher who rarely takes time to rest. For months she has felt drained. She catches every cold, gains weight despite unchanged habits, and wakes up tired no matter how long she sleeps. Her routine tests are all normal, except for one. Her cortisol curve, measured across the day, shows signs of strain: very high in the morning and flat toward evening, instead of gradually declining. This pattern tells the story of an HPA axis stuck in overdrive. High cortisol keeps her immune system suppressed, so infections linger. It changes how her body processes energy, leading to weight gain. And because the stress signal never fades, her sleep no longer restores her. In simple terms, Anna's biology behaves as though the bear never left the classroom.

Nerves in Balance: Autonomic Nervous System

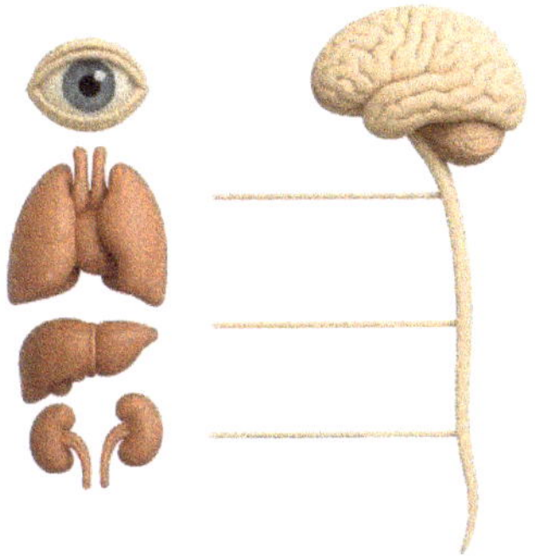

We have seen how the HPA axis sustains the long-term stress response. Now let us turn to its close partner, the autonomic nervous system (ANS). If the HPA axis governs endurance, the ANS handles moment-to-moment balance between action and rest.

It has two branches. The *sympathetic* system is the accelerator; the *parasympathetic*, the brake. In a healthy body, these two forces shift like a rhythm: effort followed by release, tension followed by repair. Under chronic stress, that rhythm begins to fail. The sympathetic drive dominates while the parasympathetic quiets. The accelerator jams; the brakes grow weak. The body stays ready for crisis even when life appears calm.

This imbalance touches nearly every organ system. The pupils stay widened, scanning for threat. The brain narrows its focus to survival, blurring concentration and disturbing sleep. The heart races with fewer natural pauses, producing palpitations and high blood pressure. Breathing becomes shallow and fast. The digestive tract loses its rhythm: the stomach rebels with reflux, the intestines with cramps and constipation. Muscles tighten, blood vessels constrict, and the body grows tense, leading to headaches, back pain, or cold hands. Even the skin mirrors the turmoil, flushing, sweating, or turning pale with every surge of stress. Meanwhile, immunity weakens while inflammation rises, creating the strange combination of frequent infections and chronic illness. All of this begins with a single signal from the brain's command center, the hypothalamus - a flicker that sets the autonomic rhythm in motion.

Case: Mark, The Accountant

Mark, a 45-year-old accountant, had spent years living in this state: racing heartbeats, unpredictable diarrhea, and restless nights. Several times he sought urgent care for crushing pain in his chest, convinced something was seriously wrong. Each investigation brought detailed reassurance: his heart was structurally sound, his lungs clear, his bloodwork unremarkable. Yet nothing eased the sense that danger was near. Mark's body had become fluent in emergency and illiterate in calm. His sympathetic system held the stage while the parasympathetic waited in silence.

When the Alarm Won't Switch Off: Central Sensitization

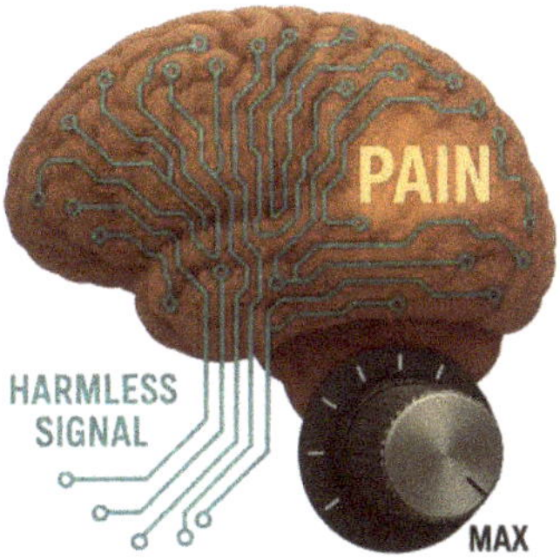

Chronic stress does not stop at hormones or the autonomic nervous system. Over time, it can reshape the central nervous system; a process called *central sensitization,* when neurons become overly reactive. Signals that are normally harmless - a light touch, a change in temperature, a faint sound - are suddenly felt as painful or overwhelming. The world grows too sharp, too loud, too much.

The mechanism lies in the sensitivity of neurons. With repeated stress or pain, nerve cells begin to fire more easily and for longer. Pain is no longer just transmitted; it is amplified. This is neuroplasticity, the nervous system's ability to learn, but in this case, it has learned a painful lesson.

Several forces reinforce this mislearning. Somatic priming, sometimes called *"wind-up,"* means that repeated pain makes nerves even more responsive. Psychobiographic shaping, or *"pain proneness,"* is a term describing how life history and personality influence pain perception. Stress load, or *"action proneness,"* keeps the whole system on high alert, ready to react before a real threat even appears. Together, they create a feedback loop that behaves as though the body is still under attack, long after the danger is gone. The result is a nervous system that has forgotten how to settle. Many people with such conditions face disbelief from employers, families, or even clinicians.

This helps explain why many patients experience severe, persistent symptoms even when MRIs, blood tests, or physical exams reveal nothing alarming. Their suffering is not imagined. They are living inside a rewired system, one that has become too good at sensing pain and too poor at finding rest. Central sensitization and hypersensitization are key mechanisms behind conditions such as fibromyalgia, chronic fatigue syndrome, migraine, neuropathic pain, and functional pain syndromes. They also underlie sensory hypersensitivities: *photophobia,* when light feels unbearable, or *phonophobia,* when ordinary sounds feel invasive.

Case: Sofia, The Young Woman with Fibromyalgia

Sofia is 29. Five years ago, she sprained her ankle while hiking. The injury healed, but the pain never truly left. Over time, it spread, first up her leg, then through her whole body. Today, even a gentle touch hurts. She wakes up tired, struggles to focus, and moves through her days as if wrapped in fog. Her doctors have ordered every test imaginable: MRIs, blood work, neurological exams… all showing healthy tissue, intact nerves, no hidden disease. Yet the pain persists, inexplicably real. What explains her suffering is central hypersensitization. After the injury, her nervous system never stood down. The pathways that once carried danger signals kept firing, becoming more excitable and reactive. Pain no longer reflected damage; it reflected a system stuck in survival mode.

When Feelings Have No Words: Alexithymia

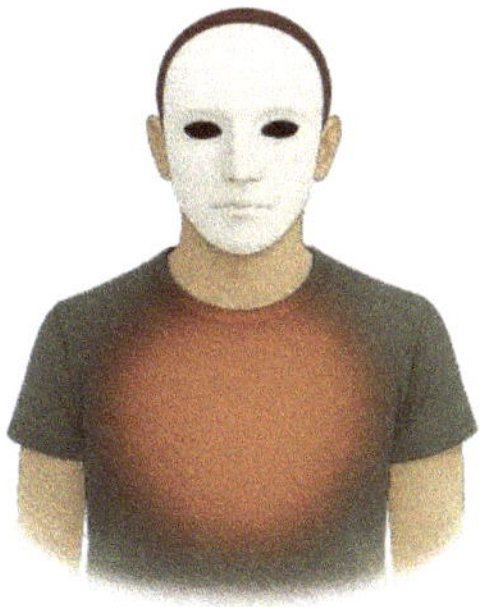

There's a word in medicine, alexithymia, that literally means "no words for emotions." It describes a difficulty in recognizing, naming, or expressing feelings, a kind of emotional unawareness. People with alexithymia often sense that something is wrong in their body but cannot link it to an inner state. The language of emotion becomes replaced by the language of symptoms.

Instead of saying *"I feel anxious,"* they might say *"my heart is racing."* Instead of recognizing sadness, they might describe a tightness in the chest or fatigue. For them, the body does the talking. This is not a lack of intelligence or willpower; it is a gap in emotional awareness, often learned early in life.

Many grew up in environments where feelings were unsafe or ignored. They learned to suppress or disconnect from their emotional world. A calm appearance doesn't always mean a calm body. Over time, this disconnection becomes automatic: feelings rise but cannot be identified, so they spill into the body. Psychologically, the emotion is muted; physiologically, it is amplified. The result is a nervous system that carries emotion as tension, pain, or exhaustion.

For clinicians, this has clear implications. Patients with alexithymia often report long lists of physical symptoms but struggle to describe their inner life. They may appear calm while their body is in turmoil. Recognizing this pattern allows us to translate and help them build a bridge between sensations and emotions, between body and mind.

Case: David, The Man with Chest Pain

David is 34. He has been to the emergency department several times with crushing chest pain. Each time, the heart tests are reassuring. His cardiovascular system is strong, his scans and labs clear. Yet the pain returns, sometimes at work, sometimes late at night. When asked about stress, David shrugs. "I don't feel stressed," he says. But his wife quietly adds that since his father's death, he has never cried, never spoken of grief, never allowed himself to feel it. What David cannot express in words, his body expresses through the chest. The pressure he never released has found a physical form. His body grieves in silence. David is not imagining his pain. He is living it, through a nervous system that has been carrying unspoken emotion for too long. Like someone who keeps running from a bear, he has learned to keep moving, suppressing every feeling that might slow him down.

Trauma Written in Molecules: Epigenetics and Trauma

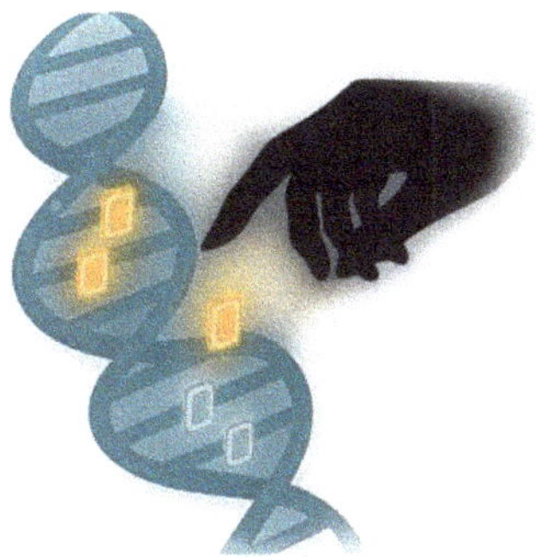

Epigenetics refers to the biological mechanisms that sit on top of our genes. They don't change the DNA itself; the letters remain the same, but they determine how strongly certain genes are expressed, like dimmer switches controlling the brightness of a light. These molecular switches guide normal development, deciding whether a cell becomes part of the brain, the skin, or the immune system.

But the same system that builds us also records us. Experience, especially stress and trauma, can leave durable marks on gene regulation. These marks don't rewrite the code; they adjust the way it's read. Studies show that early adversity is linked not only to psychological difficulties but to measurable biological changes: shifts in how the stress axis functions, higher baseline inflammation, and even subtle alterations in brain regions such as the amygdala and hippocampus, areas central to emotion and memory.

These effects can ripple across generations. When parents or grandparents have lived through chronic threat or violence, the echoes may reach their children. A mother's own early trauma can shape her physiology during pregnancy. Her hormones, immune responses, and even the composition of her blood can influence the developing stress system of the child. The biology of care and neglect thus becomes part of what families inherit, not only through behavior but through molecular memory. Early stress during sensitive windows of development can reprogram how the stress system functions, priming the brain and body for vigilance long after danger has passed. Yet the story is not fatalistic: what has been written can also be rewritten. Healing relationships, therapy, movement, rest, and small experiences of safety can shift the same switches toward recovery. The body that once learned survival can learn safety again.

Case: Leila, Heir To Unspoken Wounds

Leila is 22. Her mother grew up during years marked by fear and silence, where survival meant suppression. Her grandmother before her carried memories of flight and loss she rarely spoke of. Leila was born into this lineage of tension, through bodies that never truly exhaled. As a child she felt unease she could not name, the way her mother startled at sudden sounds or clenched her jaw when emotions rose. Now, Leila suffers from panic attacks, chronic gut pain, and a constant inner tension, though medical tests show no physical cause. Her body follows patterns older than her own life: a nervous system shaped by generations who had to stay alert. The trauma is ancestral, its residues carried through biology and behavior alike: cortisol rhythms, attachment cues, unspoken grief. Her symptoms are the body's way of remembering what her family could never fully speak or resolve.

The Clock of Our Cells: Telomeres and Aging

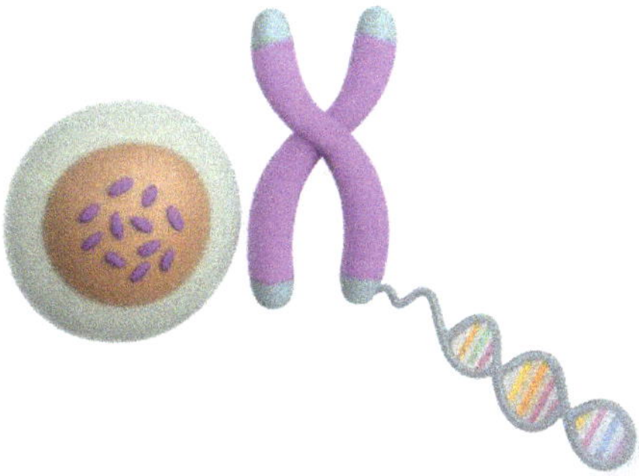

Have you ever noticed how some people seem to catch every cold, while others rarely fall ill? The difference is not only in habits or luck; it may reach down to the biology of the cell itself. At the ends of our chromosomes lie telomeres, tiny protective caps that function like the plastic tips on shoelaces. As long as those tips remain intact, the lace, our DNA, stays stable. But each time a cell divides, its telomeres shorten. When they become too short, the cell can no longer divide safely. It either stops reproducing, entering a state of cellular aging, or self-destructs through programmed cell death. This gradual shortening is part of normal aging. But when stress is chronic, the process accelerates.

Long-term exposure to stress hormones such as cortisol speeds up telomere wear, aging cells prematurely and weakening the body's defenses. Research shows clear links: childhood adversity, prolonged caregiving, and persistent emotional strain are all associated with shorter telomeres.

Why does this matter? Because telomeres do more than guard DNA ends. They influence how genes are expressed, how the immune system repairs itself, and how resilient the brain remains under stress.

The hopeful part is that telomeres are not fixed. They respond to care as much as to strain. Psychotherapy, physical activity, mindfulness, social connection, and restorative sleep all seem to stabilize telomeres, and in some studies, even lengthen them.

Case: Maria, The Caregiver

Maria is 55. For more than ten years, she cared for her husband as dementia slowly took his independence. She was cooking, washing, comforting, while her own life shrank around the illness. Now, long after his passing, Maria says she feels "twenty years older." And if you ask her biology and measure telomeres, she is. Maria's case shows what years of unrelieved caregiving stress can do: the biology of compassion turning into the biology of exhaustion. Her fatigue is not only emotional; it is cellular.

Bonds that Heal, Bonds that Hurt: Attachment Research

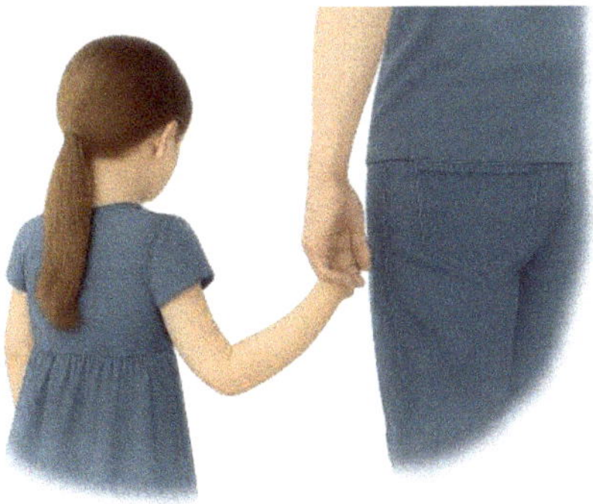

Attachment describes how humans form emotional bonds and regulate closeness and distance in relationships. It develops in early life and continues to shape how people handle stress, emotion, and connection throughout adulthood. These early patterns are not only psychological; they also leave biological and behavioral traces that affect health across the lifespan. Insecure attachment has been linked to higher physical health risks. People who grew up with inconsistent or unreliable caregivers are more likely to smoke, misuse alcohol, or struggle with weight regulation.

Attachment style also affects how patients *cope with illness*. Securely attached individuals tend to use flexible, adaptive strategies. They seek support when needed and maintain trust in the treatment process. In contrast, those with insecure attachment often rely on rigid or maladaptive strategies. This can worsen the course of chronic pain, cancer, and psychosomatic conditions. It can also complicate recovery after *medical interventions* such as organ transplantation or weight-loss surgery.

Treatment adherence is another area where attachment matters. Insecure attachment has been consistently associated with poorer adherence in chronic diseases such as diabetes, or hypertension. Secure attachment, by contrast, supports collaboration and trust, the two elements most essential for following long-term medical plans.

The *doctor-patient relationship* mirrors these dynamics. Insecurely attached patients may struggle with trust, find it difficult to regulate emotions, especially anger or shame, and bring old relational patterns into consultations.

A related concept is *mentalization*, the ability to recognize and understand one's own thoughts and emotions and those of others. Weak mentalization means that emotions are poorly understood, symptoms dominate, and relationships become sources of confusion rather than regulation. Strengthening mentalization in therapy can improve both psychological well-being and medical outcomes. Attachment, then, is not background psychology. It is a central biological and relational factor that shapes coping, health behavior, treatment adherence and the course of chronic disease.

Case: Peter, The Patient With Diabetes

Peter is 52 and lives with type 2 diabetes. Despite repeated consultations and clear treatment plans, his blood sugar remains unstable. He skips medications, ignores dietary advice, and avoids follow-up appointments. When asked why, his answers drift between irritation and helplessness. Over time, a pattern emerges. Peter describes his doctors as "cold" or "too critical." He reacts defensively in consultations, as though expecting judgment. Further exploration reveals a childhood marked by emotional distance and unpredictability. He grew up learning that closeness could not be trusted. Now, in adulthood, those early patterns reappear in the clinic. Peter's insecure attachment makes trust fragile and emotions hard to name. When overwhelmed, he withdraws or reacts with anger, instead of asking for help. His difficulties with emotion regulation and mentalization directly affect how he manages his illness.

Scars That Last: Long-Term Consequences of Early Stress

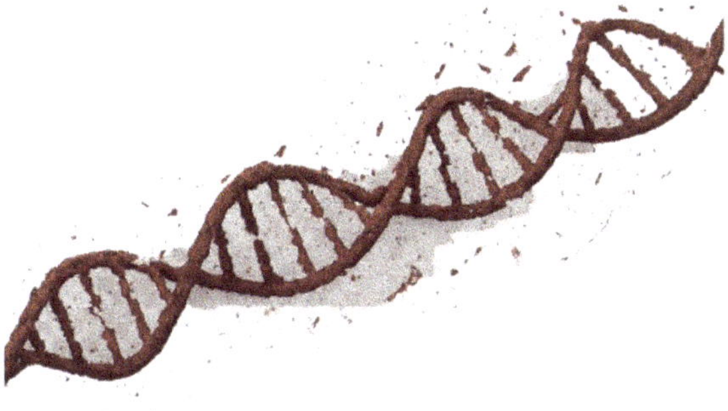

One of the most influential studies in this field, the *Adverse Childhood Experiences (ACE) Study* in the 90s, demonstrated that the accumulation of four or more early stress factors doubles or even quadruples the risk of serious adult diseases. The list is striking: type 2 diabetes, stroke, coronary heart disease, chronic lung disease, and cancers such as lung, throat or cervical cancer. Later research confirmed these findings and expanded them. Childhood adversity is linked to higher rates of cardiovascular, gastrointestinal, respiratory, metabolic, musculoskeletal and neurological conditions. It also increases the likelihood of functional syndromes such as fibromyalgia, chronic fatigue, irritable bowel syndrome, chronic widespread pain and jaw pain or dysfunction.

The effects reach beyond the body. Early stress significantly increases the risk of eating disorders, substance use, anxiety and depression. One of the most alarming findings concerns **suicidality**: individuals with multiple early stressors may face a risk of suicide attempts up to *thirty times* higher than those without! A severely burdened childhood, defined as six or more ACE factors, can shorten life expectancy by nearly *twenty years*.

Case: Amanda, The Woman With Many Illnesses

Amanda is 48. She lives with type 2 diabetes, high blood pressure, chronic back pain, irritable bowel symptoms, and frequent migraines. Despite careful medical management, she feels constantly drained. "It's as if my whole body is tired of fighting," she says. When her story is explored in depth, the thread becomes clear. Amanda grew up in a home marked by violence, unpredictability and heavy alcohol use. Her parents separated when she was six and she spent parts of her childhood in foster care. The stress of those early years shaped how her body learned to survive, always alert, always ready. Now, decades later, her biology still behaves as though the danger never ended. Her diabetes, hypertension, back pain, bowel problems and migraines are not separate illnesses, but the footprints of the same long chase.

Your Perspective, Your Practice

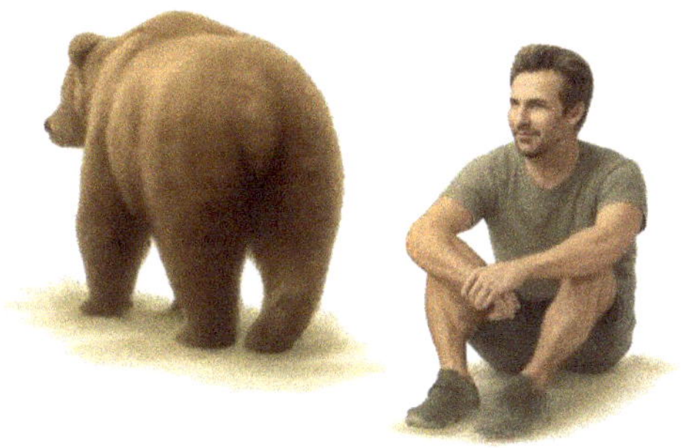

Psychosomatic symptoms are real. They are not "just in the head." They reflect measurable biological processes. These mechanisms explain why body and mind can no longer be treated as separate worlds. They are one continuous system. These patterns also live in families and systems.

This knowledge is not meant to remain theoretical. It belongs in daily clinical practice, in the small, real moments of patient care. Whether you are a general practitioner, psychiatrist, psychologist, nurse, social worker, or physiotherapist, you already meet these patients every day. They are in emergency rooms, clinics, private practices, and community health centers. Their symptoms may look purely physical, but their stories are always embodied.

Psychosomatic medicine reminds us that suffering has meaning. Life experiences are written into biology, but biology can also change again through therapy, relationships, and healing practices. Use these insights in your own way, in your own language, with your own patients. Whether through explanation, presence, or curiosity, each act of understanding helps the body remember safety again. Healing begins not when symptoms disappear, but when meaning returns.

CHAPTER TWO

Psychosomatic Assessment and Bodily Distress Disorder

How To Approach Chapter Two

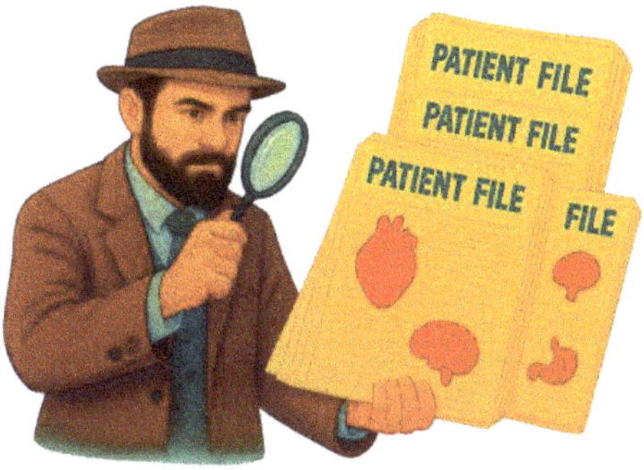

Have you ever had a headache after a stressful day at work? Most of us have. It fades with rest, and life goes on. Now imagine not just a headache, but stomach cramps, palpitations, dizziness, and fatigue; not just after work, but all the time. For weeks. For months. For years. The body feels unwell, yet tests show no disease. This is the terrain of psychosomatic medicine, where psychosomatic assessment and *Bodily Distress Disorder,* a condition in which the body shows distress without an identifiable disease, come into focus.

Even when stories are messy or emotions are hidden, people do not seek help when everything is fine. The visit itself carries meaning. Someone is asking for help, and sometimes it is a different kind of help than they expected. Think of psychosomatic assessment like a detective arriving at a scene with clues scattered everywhere. A footprint here, a broken window there, a smudge on the glass. Cramps, palpitations, or fatigue at first look unrelated, even misleading. The task is not to dismiss the evidence, but to gather them, link them and read the pattern. As the fragments connect, the picture shifts from chaos to coherence. Bodily Distress Syndrome becomes the unifying frame: a way of understanding why multiple, persistent physical symptoms cluster without a single organ disease.

And this assessment is already treatment. By treating each symptom as meaningful evidence, you validate suffering, bring structure to complexity, and open a path forward. With the right frame and tools, patients can move from confusion and fear toward clarity, regulation, and recovery.

This chapter invites you to take the role of a detective as you read.

When Symptoms Shift: Testing Change in the Interview

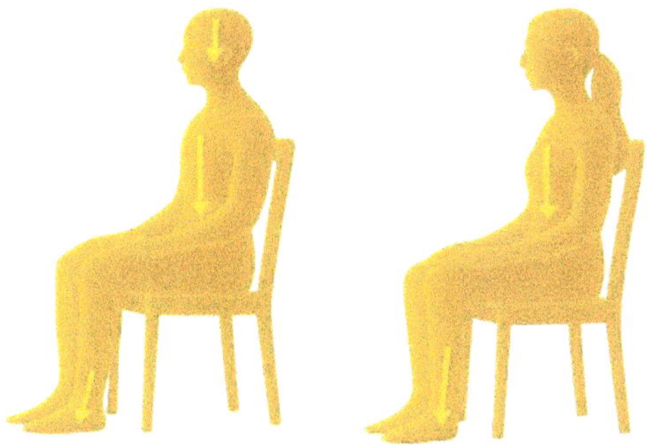

Psychosomatic assessment begins with listening and watching. Some call it "listening with your eyes." The way symptoms shift during a conversation often tells us more than any test. Many patients believe their symptoms are fixed and beyond their control, yet with careful observation, we often see them change right in front of us.

A structured *body scan* is a useful diagnostic starting point. It won't give you information with every patient, but for some, it becomes the turning point. Early in the consultation, invite the patient to notice their body slowly, from head to toe: forehead, jaw, shoulders, chest, stomach, hands, legs, and feet. Ask them to rate their main symptom: *"How strong is your headache right now, from 0 to 10?"* as they go. This anchors the number in bodily awareness. Meanwhile, you observe: a clenched jaw, raised shoulders, shallow breathing, fidgeting hands. Sometimes a sigh or a yawn appears, small signs that the nervous system is already shifting toward regulation. Next comes stress activation: ask the patient to talk about something stressful happening right now. Symptoms often rise within seconds. These shifts reveal how closely symptoms follow current emotional stress. Finally, guide a release scan. Repeat the head-to-toe process, inviting gentle relaxation. Instead, if you're experienced, you can also conduct an emotion-focused interview with the same goal.

The result varies. Some patients relax and symptoms ease. Others experience worsening. And some show no change at all. Each outcome carries diagnostic meaning and offers a moment for psychoeducation:

"You see that you can influence your symptoms yourself."
"You see that stress in this moment increases your pain."
"You see that nothing changes, as if your system is saying, 'I can't relax, I must stay alert.'"

Whichever way it goes, both clinician and patient learn something vital: the body is not static. It is a living system that reacts to stress and safety in real time. All of this happens without physical touch, only through conversation. Some patients may first need a sense of safety before focusing inward.

Case: Lara, the Curious Case (Part I: The Visit)

Lara, thirty-six, presents with a long list of complaints: daily headaches, burning in the stomach, tingling in her arms and legs, intolerance to light and sound, unpredictable fatigue, and a catalogue of supposed allergies. She describes herself as "reactive to everything." Despite multiple consultations and reassuring results, she remains convinced that something serious has been missed. At the start of the session, she rates her headache at ***7 out of 10****. Her shoulders are lifted, jaw tense, breathing shallow. Even in stillness, her body seems braced for impact. The conversation begins quietly, focused on the present moment. When asked to describe a recent stressful event, her pulse quickens, and the pain rises to* ***8****. Her voice sharpens. The activation is immediate and visible. Then comes the release scan. She follows the guidance (forehead, jaw, shoulders, breath), step by step. Gradually, the sigh appears, the breathing deepens, and the skin tone shifts. "It's less," she says, surprised. "Maybe* **5** *now." The numbers are not the point; the movement is. This is not suggestion or trickery; it is physiology rediscovering its flexibility. This moment becomes the first clue. The symptom is not fixed; it reacts to what happens within and around her. If the body changes in front of us, what exactly are we uncovering? A damaged system, or a system trying to speak?*

Looking at the Whole Picture: Somatic Assessment

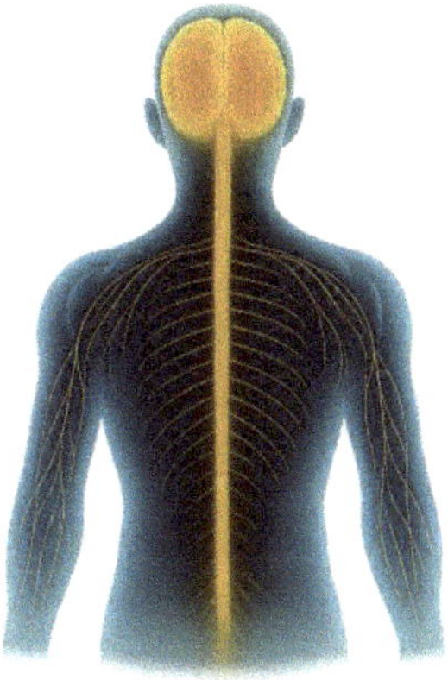

When patients come with persistent physical complaints, the first task is always a careful clinical history. Done well, it can prevent years of unnecessary referrals and countless negative tests. A practical way to think about it is in three levels.

The first level is describing the symptoms themselves. In theory, each symptom can be explored through seven dimensions: onset and course, location and quality, intensity and frequency, aggravating and relieving factors, timing, accompanying symptoms, and personal meaning. In practice, a lot of patients arrive with a long list, ten or more symptoms at once. Asking all seven questions for each would take too long. It is usually enough to focus on two or three main complaints and return to the others later. Once the picture becomes clearer, minor symptoms often fade on their own, and you don't have to assess them. Certain patterns should raise suspicion of a psychosomatic process. Symptoms that flare at night or on waking, that persist long after an injury has healed, or that worsen with emotional conflict are all clues. Complaints that do not follow anatomical pathways, that shift from one body part to another or are triggered by light, sound, weather, or food, also point in this direction. Many patients have long histories of functional disorders such as irritable bowel syndrome, fibromyalgia, chronic fatigue, migraine, or overlapping anxiety and depression.

The second level is the physical examination and medical exclusion. Our first duty is to rule out dangerous disease. This means a thorough general exam: vital signs, chest, abdomen, musculoskeletal system and a brief neurological screen. Basic laboratory work typically includes blood count, inflammation markers, thyroid function, glucose, kidney and liver profile. Imaging is often used, especially for headaches, back pain, or joint complaints, but it should follow clinical reasoning, not routine. These tests confirm the body's hardware is intact before we look at its wiring. Red flags such as weight loss, bleeding, or neurological deficits always justify further testing. Yet many scans reveal incidental findings, like mild disc protrusions, small cysts or age-related changes, that may explain little. A "positive" result does not rule out psychosomatic factors; it simply adds another layer to interpret.

The third level is the biopsychosocial history. This widens the lens. Biological: medical history, medications, lifestyle, sleep, nutrition, family risk factors… Psychological: stress reactivity, coping style, emotional awareness (alexithymia), trauma history… Social: relationships, work stress, financial strain, cultural context, available support… When these levels are combined, symptoms begin to make sense.

Case: Lara, the Curious Case (Part II: The Traces)

On some days her hands feel numb; on others, her chest burns. She has tried elimination diets, antihistamines, magnesium, and physiotherapy. Nothing helps for long. "It's like my body keeps inventing new ways to fail," she says. Her symptoms do not follow anatomical pattern. Tingling alternates sides. The burning shifts from stomach to skin. The pain sometimes wakes her at night and eases when she is distracted. These fluctuations already suggest a functional process, but the assessment must still be thorough. Vital signs are stable. Neurological and musculoskeletal exams are without focal deficits. Laboratory results are within normal limits. An earlier MRI had shown only minor age-related changes. The evidence rules out acute disease but confirms nothing about cause. The biopsychosocial history starts to connect the fragments. Biologically, Lara eats irregularly, sleeps poorly, and relies on painkillers and antihistamines. Psychologically, she describes herself as calm but admits that anger "doesn't fit" her. When tension rises, she withdraws or goes numb. Socially, she works in a demanding open-plan office and spends her evenings caring for her mother, who has chronic illness. She feels guilty when resting, anxious when stopped. Each layer adds coherence. Her symptoms are not random; they trace the contours of a life under strain. The question is no longer where the illness sits, but how her system keeps the alarm switched on. If every test reassures but the body remains distressed, what keeps the signal alive? Faulty organs, or a body that has learned to stay alert?

Measuring the Invisible: Structured Diagnostic Tools

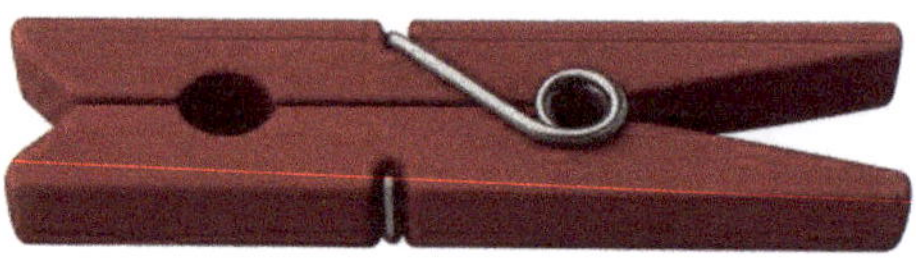

After the clinical history and physical examination, we can go one step further and use *structured tools*. These do not replace listening to the patient, but they help organize complexity, measure severity and track progress. Not every clinician needs them, and not every patient benefits from them. For some, a good conversation and clinical intuition are enough. But for those who appreciate structure, these tools can become a powerful part of the process. They make symptoms visible, change measurable, and explanations concrete. Sometimes, they even open difficult conversations that might not have started otherwise.

The first tool is **pressure pain threshold testing**, in Switzerland often done with the *Algopeg* (Egloff et al.). The device looks like a clothes peg but is calibrated to 10 newtons. It is applied to both middle fingers and both earlobes, and the patient rates the pain after 10 seconds on a scale from 0 to 10. Research shows that this simple device correlates well with electronic algometers. High sensitivity points toward central sensitization, but also unusually low pain responses may reflect altered perception. The advantage is clear: it is quick, reliable, inexpensive, and easy to repeat in daily practice. In psychosomatic assessment, it provides a bridge between subjective experience and measurable physiology. It's a concrete way to show that hypersensitivity is real.

Then comes the **pain drawing**. Patients mark their symptoms directly on a body outline: red for pain, blue for sensations such as tingling or cold. This makes vague or diffuse complaints concrete, especially when words are hard to find. The drawings often reveal patterns that do not follow dermatomes or anatomical structures, suggesting a functional explanation. But they can also point toward organic processes: symmetric joint involvement may suggest a rheumatologic condition, while glove-and-stocking distributions may indicate neuropathy. For many patients, this simple visual exercise becomes the first time they "see" their own symptoms in front of them.

Beyond physical measures, structured **questionnaires** can add another layer of understanding. The Patient Health Questionnaire-15 (PHQ-15) sketches the weight of physical symptoms, while the Somatic Symptom Disorder-12 (SSD-12) gives a glimpse into the mental echo: the worry, the rumination, the pull these thoughts can have on daily life. The Hospital Anxiety and Depression Scale (HADS) adds a layer, tracing the anxiety and low mood that so often travel beside bodily distress. There are other questionnaires as well, which I won't list here, that capture daily strain and bodily awareness, offering a broader view beyond symptoms alone. Finally, there are separate questionnaires that explore life history and personality patterns. The **Adverse Childhood Experiences (ACE)** questionnaire helps identify early trauma, which often increases later vulnerability. But timing matters. Giving the ACE too early can overwhelm patients. Some withdraw if it arrives too soon. In my experience, it works best when completed together, once a stable alliance has formed, so that the answers can be understood in context. Simple **trait checklists** for perfectionism, self-criticism, or over-adaptation can reveal patterns that keep stress high.

Used thoughtfully, these instruments do not replace the clinical encounter, they deepen it.

Case: Lara, the Curious Case (Part III: The Evidence)

*Lara agrees to continue the assessment. She sits upright, cautious but curious. The Algopeg test begins. Pressure on her middle fingers registers **6 out of 10**, already higher than most people. When applied to her earlobes, she flinches and pulls away after three seconds. "That's unbearable," she says, rating it **10 out of 10**. On the pain drawing, she marks her knees and lower abdomen in red, her hands and feet in blue. The map is diffuse, crossing anatomical borders, a trace of constant alarm rather than injury. The questionnaires confirm the pattern: high somatic burden, strong emotional preoccupation,* *exhaustion from vigilance itself. When offered the ACE questionnaire, she insists on completing it right away. She moves through it quickly, answering 'no' to every question, her tone flat, her gaze distant. The topic is left untouched for now. Each layer adds meaning. Her sensitivity is real, her defenses strong, her story still guarded. If the body protects against even gentle touch, and the mind closes against memory, what kind of understanding could reach them both?*

Connecting the Dots: Diagnosing Bodily Distress Disorder

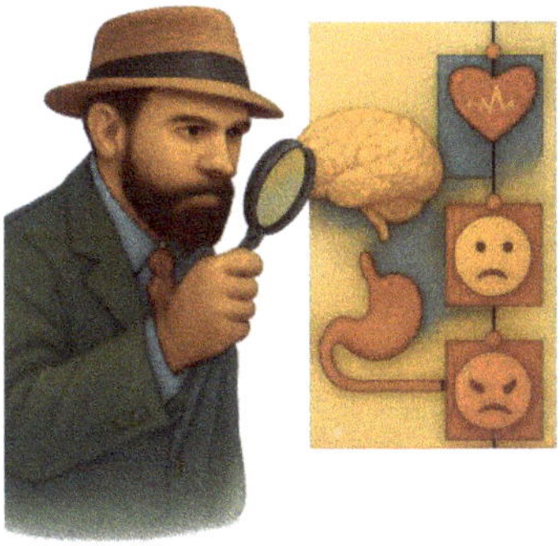

After the clinical history, physical examination, and structured tools comes the most delicate part of psychosomatic assessment: bringing everything together. This is where scattered clues turn into a story.

In ICD-11 (section 6C20), this coherent picture is called Bodily Distress Disorder (BDD), closely related to what research traditions describe as Bodily Distress Syndrome (BDS). Both describe the same phenomenon: a system under chronic strain, where the body speaks when words cannot. The diagnostic criteria are straightforward, but their interpretation is an art. Symptoms tend to gather in four clusters: cardiopulmonary (palpitations, chest pain, or shortness of breath), gastrointestinal (abdominal pain, bloating, diarrhea, or nausea), musculoskeletal (muscle pain, joint pain, or back pain); and general and fatigue-related (dizziness, exhaustion, or concentration problems). Many patients have symptoms spanning at least three clusters, but others may have a single dominant complaint, chronic pain, persistent fatigue, or one organ system that never seems to recover.

The core features are duration (months or years), how much daily life is affected, and the lack of a better medical explanation. When all the pieces align, we see a pattern, one that can be explained and shared with the patient. This is why BDS is not a diagnosis of exclusion. It is a diagnosis of integration. It does not say *"nothing is wrong."* It says, *"here is how the parts fit together."*

Case: Lara, the Curious Case (Part IV: The Verdict)

When the pieces are placed side by side, the picture comes into focus. Lara's symptoms fall into three clear clusters: gastrointestinal, musculoskeletal, and fatigue-related. Each has persisted for years, each limits her daily life, and none can be explained by structural disease. Together they form the recognizable pattern of ***Bodily Distress Syndrome,*** *a body that remains in defense long after the threat is gone. Explaining this is delicate. The word psychosomatic can sound to patients like imaginary, yet it means something far more grounded: that body and mind operate as one system. Lara listens quietly as the findings are laid out: the heightened sensitivity, the fluctuating pain, the nervous system reacting as though danger were always near. When the logic becomes clear, she exhales for the first time that day. "So it's real," she says. "Just... not the way I thought." The diagnosis gives her a frame, not a label. It opens a path for treatment, and for understanding. The body had never been lying; it had been speaking in the only language it knew.*

Calming the Body First: Body-Oriented Interventions

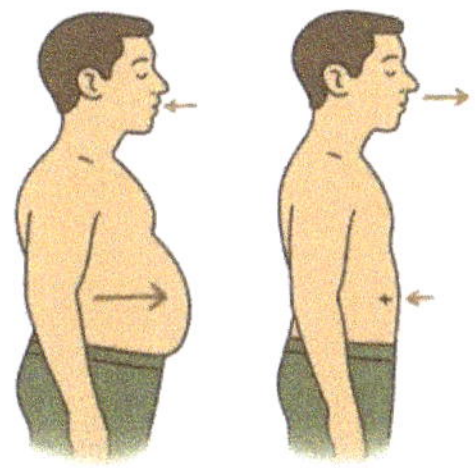

Once patients begin to speak about their suffering, we don't need to wait for a final diagnosis to help. In psychosomatic medicine, self-regulation tools can be introduced from the very first consultation. These simple exercises calm the nervous system, reduce stress, and give patients back a sense of control over their own body. Sometimes they are not only therapeutic but also diagnostic: when symptoms shift in the moment, they reveal how closely body and emotion are linked. These methods strengthen interoceptive awareness and autonomic flexibility.

A **body scan** invites the patient to move attention slowly from head to toe. Whenever possible, it should be done in detail. At first, you might offer options to help them find words: *Do you see clearly, or do you notice black dots, blurriness, tunnel vision? Does the chest feel tight or hollow? Are the hands warm or cold?* Gradually, patients learn to describe sensations on their own, in precise language rather than broad terms like "fine" or "bad." This practice builds awareness and curiosity. Instead of fear (*"What if this pain means something dangerous?"*), the focus turns to observation (*"This is warmth. This is tension. This is tingling."*). The body becomes less threatening, less foreign. Even a few minutes of guided attention can show that sensations are not fixed but constantly shifting, and that noticing them already begins to change them.

Diaphragmatic breathing is one of the fastest ways to activate the parasympathetic system, the body's natural brake. Breathing deeply into the belly, inhaling for about four seconds and exhaling slowly for six to eight, settles the heart rate and calms the mind within minutes. It is physiology, not suggestion. You can also use this technique for psychoeducation if symptoms change (described in **Section One** of this chapter).

In **progressive muscle relaxation**, patients gently tense and release muscle groups one by one. This rhythm of contraction and release teaches them to recognize tension before it builds and to let it go deliberately. Over time, the baseline stress level drops; the nervous system learns that relaxation is safe. One way to explain this neurobiologically is covered in **Chapter four**.

And when stress or panic strikes suddenly, **grounding techniques** help patients return to the present. By focusing on simple sensory details, such as the floor under the feet, the chair beneath them, or five things they can see or name, they re-anchor awareness in the body and the here and now. Dissociation and anxiety often ease within seconds. These exercises also complement physical rehabilitation and can be supported in daily routines or social settings, helping patients integrate regulation into ordinary life.

These tools are not side treatments. They are frontline methods. They can be used from the first consultation, sometimes to calm and sometimes to clarify. They show that body and mind are flexible and open to change. This is precisely why psychotherapy is so effective in psychosomatic practice.

If symptoms can shift in a few minutes of guided regulation, imagine what can happen in the structured, safe frame of ongoing therapy. What begins as small fluctuations in the consultation can become lasting change, as the nervous system learns, session by session, that it no longer needs to live in survival mode. These methods may seem simple, but they are often the turning point. They show that change is not theoretical; it is happening right now.

Case: Alina, the Teacher with Leg Pain

Alina, a teacher in her late thirties, has lived with pain in her right leg ever since an injury ten years ago. The fracture healed long ago, yet the pain remained. Painkillers bring brief relief, but the pressure always returns. During one session, she learns diaphragmatic breathing. She begins with her pain rated at 6 out of 10. For five minutes, she practices: inhaling for four seconds, exhaling for six. Gradually, her shoulders drop, her breathing deepens, and her face softens. The pain eases to 3 out of 10. This can also be diagnostic, like the body scan, but it's usually done for relaxing the system and then for psychoeducation.

Sharing the Map: Psychoeducation

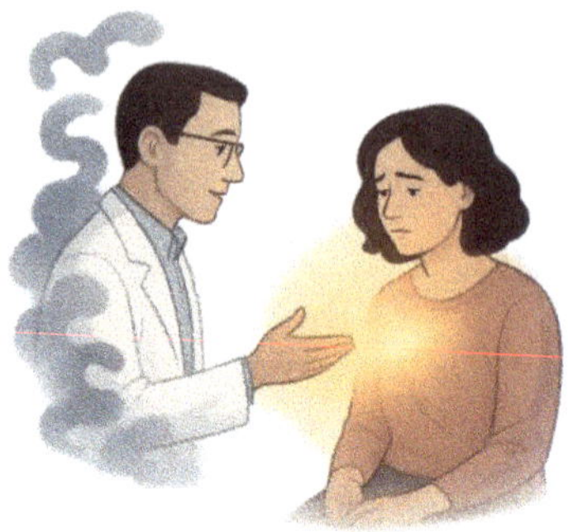

The way we explain a diagnosis often matters more than the label itself. For many patients, this conversation is the true turning point and the moment they move from fear and confusion to clarity and hope. It explains that stress and emotions can activate learned neural pathways that the brain can unlearn. It is a therapeutic intervention in itself. Patients with psychosomatic symptoms frequently carry a hidden fear of being told that "psychosomatic" means their suffering is imaginary, or worse, that they are "crazy." If that fear is not addressed directly, it poisons trust. The consultation that could heal instead becomes another injury.

The key lies not just in *what* we say, but in *how* we say it. The explanation must validate the patient's experience, ground it in biology, and open a door toward recovery. This reframe dissolves shame and opens the way to healing. Not every patient needs long-term therapy. Some improve after just two or three consultations. For them, psychoeducation alone can break the cycle. For others, psychoeducation becomes the foundation for further treatment. It can open the way to physiotherapy, relaxation training, occupational therapy, nutritional guidance, social support, biofeedback and/or psychotherapy.

When symptoms are still new, early psychoeducation can prevent chronicity. This is where general practitioners play a crucial role. They are often the first to meet these patients. A short, well-framed explanation in the early phase can save years of unnecessary suffering.

Explain it in a way that truly makes sense to you first; only then can it make sense to the patient. Studies show that clear explanations reduce repeat Emergency Room visits for functional disorders.

Case: Thomas, the Frequent Emergency Room Visitor

Thomas, 40, has been to the emergency department more times than he can count. Each visit begins the same way: crushing chest pain, dizziness, exhaustion; and every time the tests show no signs of disease. ECGs, bloodwork, cardiac imaging, all clear. Still, the fear returns. Convinced that something has been missed, he often asks to stay for observation, only to leave more anxious than before. One day, a doctor in the ER does something different. She doesn't order more tests. She offers an image to help him understand. She sits down and says, "Your heart is healthy. Your lungs are fine. What's happening is that your body's alarm system has become too sensitive. Imagine there was once a fire in this office. The alarm went off, the sprinklers started, and the fire was put out. To make sure it never happens again, we turn the alarm sensitivity to high, so it reacts sooner next time. Maybe there will never be another fire, but we do it out of precaution. The problem is that now, even a little smoke from the kitchen sets it off. Water sprays everywhere, soaking everything, and it becomes impossible to work. Your body's alarm works like that. It once protected you when you needed it most, but now it reacts too quickly, creating chaos instead of safety. What we can do is help that alarm return to a more balanced setting. You still need it, just not this sensitive. And we can look at how to protect what really matters so that your system feels safe again." For Thomas, this explanation changes everything. For the first time, the story of his suffering makes sense. He leaves the ER calmer, with a sense that there is a path forward and that with the right guidance, he can learn to retrain his alarm system.

Not Everything Is Psychosomatic

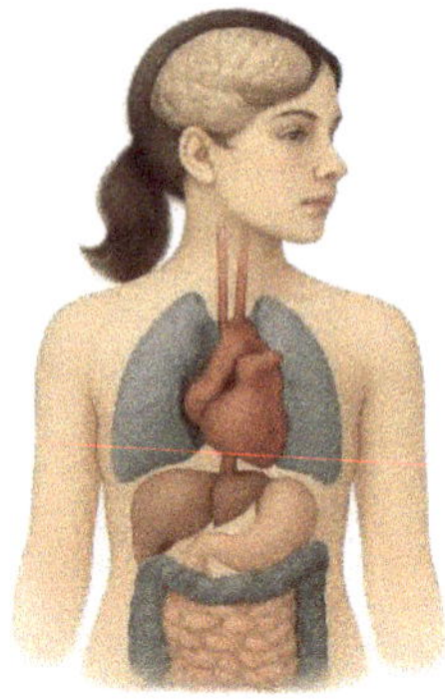

If a patient doesn't get better, it may not be a resistant case, but an unsolved one. Psychosomatic medicine teaches us how deeply the mind and body intertwine. But sometimes, what looks psychosomatic at first hides something entirely different. The same empathy that hears emotion in the body must also keep an eye open for biology. The best clinicians are those who can hold both lenses at once: to know when to look deeper into the psyche and when to look again into the blood, the genes, or the cells.

Some conditions, especially in their early stages, can look psychosomatic but are not. *Multiple sclerosis* may begin with vague sensations like numbness, weakness, or blurred vision that come and go. *Systemic lupus erythematosus* often brings fatigue, joint pain, mood swings, and shifting skin changes. *Celiac disease* can hide behind abdominal pain, exhaustion, or even neurological complaints. *Lyme disease* may present as joint pain, mental slowing, or persistent fatigue. *Addison's disease* can show up as dizziness, stomach discomfort, and unexplained weight loss. *Porphyria* sometimes appears as recurrent abdominal pain mixed with psychiatric or neurological symptoms. Each of these illnesses can mimic the complexity of psychosomatic disorders. The task is not to suspect one or the other too quickly, but to hold both possibilities in mind until the pattern becomes clear.

Case: Crawling Beneath the Skin

Mira, 34, arrived exhausted and terrified. "There are worms crawling under my skin," she said. At first, it sounded like metaphor, the vivid imagery patients often use when describing tingling or itching. Perhaps it was a psychosomatic expression of distress, perhaps an anxiety disorder. But Mira's conviction was unwavering. She traced the paths the "worms" took across her arms and legs, describing in detail how they "entered" her body. Reassurance had no effect. This was not a figure of speech; it was a fixed belief. After a thorough investigation, the puzzle was resolved: Mira's suffering was not psychosomatic, but part of a psychotic disorder. At first, her story looked like a false lead, the kind of case that seems symbolic until you look closer. Psychotic disorders that haven't become chronic are treatable and not signs of moral weakness.

***Treatment:** She was started on antipsychotic medication alongside psychoeducation and social support. The task was no longer to interpret sensations but to treat the psychosis that created them.*

Case: The Depression That Wasn't Alone

Mateo, 28, came with months of low mood, hopelessness, and fatigue. He had tried antidepressants before; they helped briefly, then stopped helping and even made it worse. His symptoms fit the pattern of a depressive episode, perhaps with psychosomatic fatigue layered on top. But a detail emerged in passing: years earlier, during university, Mateo had experienced sleepless nights, boundless energy, fast speech, and reckless spending. At the time, he thought it was "just a phase." In reality, it was hypomania. A forgotten detail from years before turned out to be the missing piece of evidence. His current depression wasn't isolated; it was the low in a bipolar cycle.

***Treatment:** A mood stabilizer was introduced, and Mateo began psychoeducation on recognizing early warning signs and maintaining regular rhythms.*

Case: The Shifting Story

Semir, 35, presented with abdominal pain, mood swings, and constant crises in relationships. His complaints varied wildly, severe one week, gone the next. It looked like psychosomatic instability, the body echoing an overwhelmed mind. But the timing didn't add up. Over time, a pattern emerged: his worst crises aligned with episodes of substance use and withdrawal. His symptoms were not psychosomatic but addiction-related, shaped by both intoxication and its aftermath. The shame stopped him giving all the information.

***Treatment:** Semir entered a program for detoxification, relapse prevention, and counseling. The focus shifted from analyzing his "stress reactions" to rebuilding abstinence.*

Case: The Attacks That Left No Trace

Elena, 42, had endured years of unexplained attacks: sharp abdominal pain, fatigue, and confusion. Every test, including blood work, endoscopy and imaging, showed no abnormalities. She was told again and again it must be psychosomatic. But Elena noticed something: during attacks, her urine turned dark. One day, during an episode, a doctor ordered specialized tests. The answer appeared: acute intermittent porphyria, a rare metabolic disorder. Why did it escape detection? Routine tests between attacks often show no disease; only targeted testing during an acute episode or DNA testing reveals the truth. Years of investigation yielded nothing until one sharp-eyed doctor ordered the right test at the right moment, revealing the final clue.

Treatment: *Elena received intravenous hemin and was taught to avoid known triggers. With proper management, the attacks ceased. What had been dismissed as psychosomatic was, in fact, a rare but serious disease.*

Each story began as a potential psychosomatic case: Mira's crawling worms, Mateo's unshakable depression, Semir's chaotic symptoms, Elena's mysterious attacks. But each unfolded differently, into psychosis, bipolar disorder, addiction, and porphyria. Each demanded a distinct treatment, and each reminds us that psychosomatic thinking must never replace medical curiosity. At the same time, psychosomatic mechanisms can accompany any of these conditions: Mira may still feel bodily distress, Mateo's mood disorder may bring functional fatigue, Semir's withdrawal may amplify pain, Elena's rare illness may provoke anxiety and hypervigilance. Psychosomatic and organic processes are not enemies; they often coexist, amplifying one another. The art of medicine is to discern which dominates, and when. Even when organic disease is found, rehabilitation remains crucial to retrain body perception and movement confidence. Medicine begins to lose its soul the moment it chooses sides between body and mind.

Your Perspective, Your Practice

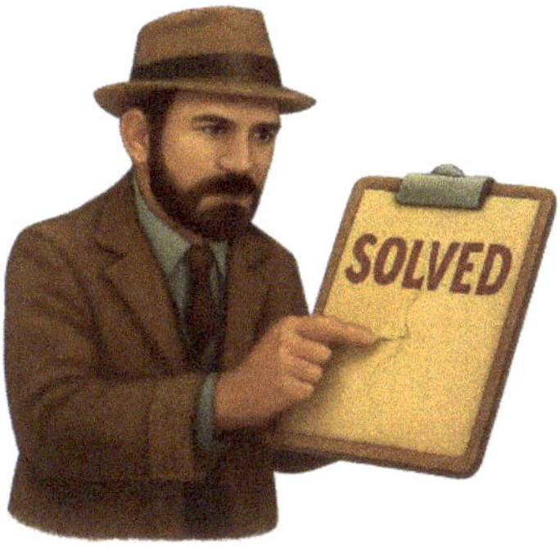

Every time you sit with a patient, you are doing more than gathering information; you are shaping an experience of care. Even before any prescription, referral, or test result, your presence already matters. That is the quiet power of your role. You are not only a part of the system. You are also a witness, a guide, and sometimes the first person to show that healing is possible. In the rush of a full clinic, this can be easy to forget, but listening itself is medicine.

This is where hope begins to grow. And hope, in psychosomatic work, is not decoration or comfort; it is often the very first physiological step toward recovery. So approach each encounter as an opportunity. This is your art. It lies in how you look, listen, and respond, in how you help patients find coherence where there was only confusion. You stand at the intersection of biology, psychology, and humanity. And in that meeting point, with each patient, you have the chance to turn fear into clarity and isolation into understanding.

Empathy is powerful, but it needs form to stay effective; without boundaries, it burns out instead of healing. Sometimes care means not only listening, but showing that help exists beyond this room, through colleagues, teams, and systems that hold the patient together when one person cannot. Hope often begins there, in the shared act of coordinated care. Because in the end, science alone cannot heal; it needs humanity to work.

You know, deep down, why you chose this kind of work. Something in you was drawn to mystery, to tracing what hides beneath the surface, to making sense where others see chaos. That instinct to look closer and listen longer is what makes you good at this. Don't forget it when the days blur and you are on the edge. Perhaps something in your story drew you to this path, but once you begin the work, motive turns into craft. You chose to be a detective, so be it.

CHAPTER THREE

Starting Psychotherapy

How To Approach Chapter Three

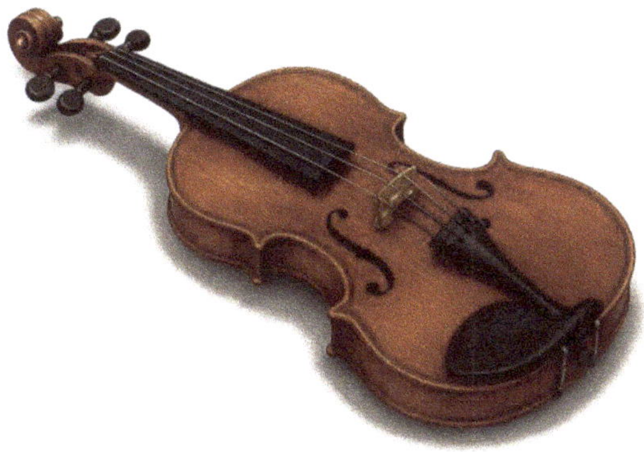

A violin must be tuned before you can play. Even a master's hands can't draw music from strings that are too tight or too loose. The wood needs warmth, the bow needs balance, and the player has to listen to the faint hum that tells them when the tone is right. Once tuned, the same four strings can produce an endless range of feeling.

Psychotherapy works much the same way. But before melody, comes tuning. Before deep work can begin, the mind and body should find balance. Structured approaches such as cognitive-behavioral therapy (CBT) and/or medication often play a big role in this preparatory phase. They help reduce noise, ease symptoms, and create the conditions where the inner strings can resonate instead of distort. Sometimes life circumstances must settle before therapy can resonate. Body awareness, movement, and human connection all help retune the instrument.

For some patients, this tuning is enough. CBT becomes their music, a daily practice that keeps their instrument in tune, helping them live with rhythm, discipline, and steadiness. Their melodies are simple, but they play a wonderful sound. For others, tuning is only the prelude. Once stability returns, they long for something fuller: to explore the emotional themes behind the notes. Deeper therapies, like schema therapy or other relational and emotion-focused methods are like playing full compositions: they uncover buried harmonies, revisit old motifs and resolve dissonances that have echoed for years. And then there are patients who arrive with years of therapy already behind them. They know the scales, the exercises, even fragments of songs, but the violin never quite sang. In these cases, the task isn't to start over, but to listen again. To retune the strings, to help them find resonance and to guide the music that was always waiting beneath the noise.

This chapter takes you from tuning the strings to enjoying the concert.

Tuning The Strings: The Role Of Medication

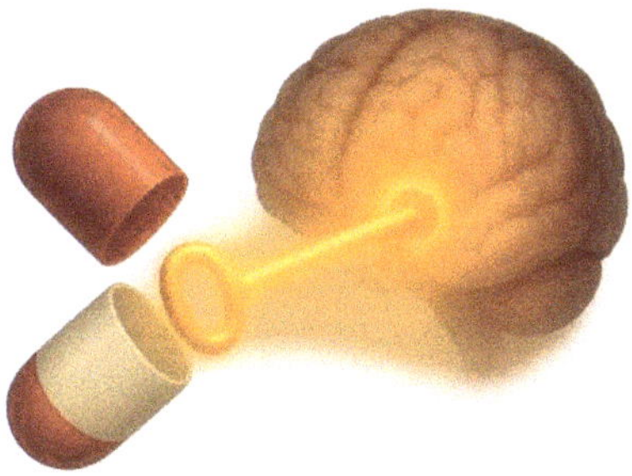

When patients arrive with psychosomatic symptoms, it's tempting to reach for the prescription pad. Medication is concrete, visible, and fast. But here's the essential principle: psychotherapy should always begin in parallel. Medication alone is never the answer. What it can do is stabilize the system, improve sleep, reduce anxiety, lift mood, or sharpen concentration. That way, patients are able to engage in therapy. And when patients are skeptical about psychotherapy, medication can buy time.

The best results often come when people talk to each other about the patient, not around them. When the prescriber, therapist, and others share what they see, treatment starts to sound like one voice instead of many scattered notes. Sometimes that also means helping the patient find what's affordable and tolerable, so the plan fits real life, not just the textbook. In psychosomatic medicine, medication is best understood as supportive, not curative. It lowers the background noise so the real work, psychotherapy, can begin.

Antidepressants such as SSRIs or SNRIs don't just treat depression; they also calm the overactive stress response, ease anxiety and sometimes reduce chronic pain. Short-term **anxiolytics** can interrupt acute crises, though always with caution about dependency. **Sleep aids** may help restore rest early on but should be paired with sleep hygiene and withdrawn as soon as stability returns. **Pain medication** can build trust in the beginning, offering relief that allows patients to stay in treatment, but it should never become the central strategy. **Herbal preparations** can be useful for those who prefer "natural" options. St. John's Wort has evidence for mild to moderate depression, while valerian or lavender can support sleep and anxiety. These are not risk-free, especially St. John's Wort, which interacts with many drugs. But when used carefully, they can help patients feel heard instead of dismissed.

Case: Julia, Major Depression (ICD-11)

Julia, 42, came with constant fatigue, body aches and a heavy sense of hopelessness. She had lost interest in everything she once enjoyed, struggled to concentrate and often lay awake at night, caught in guilt and rumination. For weeks, even getting out of bed had become a daily battle. Looking through ICD-11 information, she met the criteria for a major depressive episode. At first, therapy felt impossible. "It's useless," Julia said. "I can't even get dressed; how should I work on my thoughts?" Starting an SSRI brought her sleep back, softened her anxiety and gave her just enough energy to attend weekly sessions. With the system steadied, she began her first CBT steps: writing down thoughts, testing small behavioral experiments and slowly re-engaging with life. For the first time, Julia didn't drop out after three weeks. She stayed. And gradually, she learned how to prevent future major depressive episodes. The medication doesn't fix the story, but it tunes the instrument so that therapy can play.

Changing Thoughts, Changing Symptoms: Cognitive Behavioral Therapy

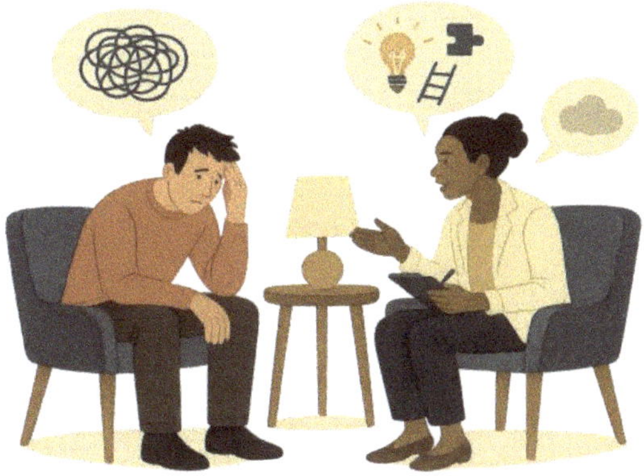

Cognitive Behavioral Therapy (CBT) is often the most effective entry point for psychotherapy in psychosomatic medicine. Its guiding principle is simple yet powerful: thoughts shape emotions and emotions shape the body. When unhelpful thoughts dominate, they generate fear. Fear activates the stress system, which in turn produces more symptoms. These symptoms then reinforce the fearful thoughts and very quickly a vicious circle forms. CBT interrupts this loop. Patients learn to observe their automatic thoughts, test them against reality, and adopt perspectives that are more balanced and useful. At the same time, they practice new behaviors that reduce avoidance, build confidence, and calm the nervous system. The goal is not immediate symptom elimination, but the gradual development of healthier patterns.

Some disorders often overlap in psychosomatic medicine, and it's hard to distinguish them. The therapeutic focus, however, remains the same: reducing fear and restoring agency. You don't necessarily need to have a diagnosis, just the right way of thinking. You can always look at the criteria and define an ICD-11 diagnosis, but that is not the point of your work here. Some diagnoses should be given after two years of therapy, so don't stress yourself with it at the beginning.

In psychosomatic medicine, certain CBT methods have proven especially valuable. *Cognitive restructuring* helps patients reframe catastrophic interpretations and test them against evidence. *Behavioral activation and exposure* counter the withdrawal that deepens symptoms, encouraging gradual re-engagement with feared or avoided situations. *Mindfulness and meditation* allow sensations to be observed without judgment, reducing the grip of fear. *Self-compassion* softens harsh inner voices and strengthens the capacity to comfort the vulnerable self. *Practical adjustments* such as setting boundaries, balancing workload, and improving sleep and movement help regulate the stress system. Thought patterns can shift muscular tone, breathing rhythm, and even posture, so each cognitive change finds an echo in the body. Each of these methods builds stability from both sides: thought and body, mind and behavior.

Among CBT-based tools, **expressive writing** deserves special mention. It is particularly useful for patients who over-intellectualize or for those with ADHD who often struggle to distinguish between thoughts and feelings. Emotions are not processed through thinking; they move through the body. Writing helps them find a channel. Patients are invited to write for 10–15 minutes daily, first their thoughts, then their feelings. You can give a patient an example: *"I went to the psychiatrist today and I was angry with him"*. When finished writing, the page is destroyed. This last step matters the most; by discarding what was written, patients learn that emotions can be expressed fully and then released rather than stored. As therapy progresses, the exercise expands. Letters are written to significant figures from past and present, parents, partners, friends, and then destroyed (maybe burnt). The practice builds the ability to face emotion honestly and to let go when its time has passed.

Case: Markus, Generalized Anxiety Disorder (ICD-11)

Markus, 41, spent most of his days caught in a loop of worry. His mind jumped from one possible disaster to the next, from bills to health to work and family, each thought tightening his chest until it felt as if something were wrong with his heart. Nights offered no rest; sleep slipped away to "what if" thoughts that grew louder in the dark. Although every medical checkup showed his body was healthy, his mind remained on alert, certain that danger was always just ahead. According to ICD-11, he met the criteria for Generalized Anxiety Disorder (GAD). When treatment began, he started with liquid medication, taking only a few drops at first because he was afraid of side effects. It took months to reach the therapeutic dose, and during that time, cognitive-behavioral therapy became his anchor. CBT gave him tools to manage the worry while the medication slowly took effect, helping him regain small pieces of daily life even before the full pharmacological benefit appeared. In CBT, Markus learned to identify catastrophic thoughts, test them against evidence and break his avoidance cycle. He practiced diaphragmatic breathing to calm his body, tracked symptoms to spot patterns and gradually reintroduced activities he had abandoned out of fear. The chest pain didn't disappear completely, but it lost its power to dominate his life.

Case: Hana, Health Anxiety Disorder (ICD-11)

Hana, 36, presented a different picture. She interpreted ordinary sensations like mild headache, stomach cramp or a flutter in the chest as signs of serious illness. She spent hours checking her body, searching online and seeking reassurance from doctors. Despite no abnormal results, her anxiety persisted. According to ICD-11, she met the criteria for Health Anxiety Disorder. Since the focus is on fear of disease, not the symptoms themselves, it doesn't fit to Bodily Distress Syndrom, nor to Generalized Anxiety Disorder. In CBT, the focus was on breaking the reassurance cycle. Hana practiced delaying body checks, reducing online searches and gradually tolerating uncertainty. Step by step, she learned to see minor sensations as part of ordinary life, rather than evidence of a catastrophe. Over time, her anxiety eased, and her life became less dominated by health fears.

Voices in Two Chairs: Schema Therapy and the Chair Technique

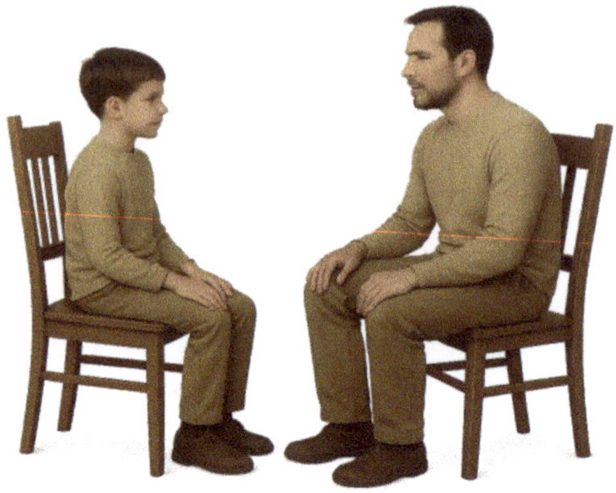

Schema therapy is a rich and complex method, but even its simplest form can offer remarkable insight. What follows is a simplified version you can use directly in psychosomatic practice. It is not full schema therapy, which requires years of training, supervision, and experience, but a focused exercise to help patients begin hearing the different parts of themselves. Even this brief version, *"two chairs and two voices"*, can reveal aspects of a patient's inner world that no test or questionnaire ever could.

This is my suggestion for you to try. Set up two chairs facing each other. One represents the child mode, the other the adult mode. If possible, use a chair with a higher back for the child's chair, so it feels like one. The patient begins in the child chair, connecting with the feelings of their younger self. It's not about inventing a story but noticing what arises naturally when they allow themselves to sit there. Then they move to the adult chair: the grounded, responsible part of themselves that can offer safety and care, and that is often weak. Strong emotions often surface during this exercise; that is not a sign of harm but of depth. They can, and should, be discussed safely within the therapeutic frame. You invite them to observe the contrast: how their body feels, how their voice changes, what emotions appear in each position. The difference itself often teaches more than any explanation. When the child doesn't trust the adult, that's not a failure; it's information. If adults were unsafe or inconsistent in childhood, the inner child will naturally distrust the adult self now. It shows how deeply trust was broken and how much work must go into rebuilding it.

Making this visible opens the way for psychoeducation about self-trust and emotional regulation. For many patients, that recognition becomes a turning point: instead of reacting from the wounded child, they begin responding from the adult self. And if these small exercises help, you can refer a patient to a schema therapy specialist.

Case: Sara, The Thin Woman (Part I: Setting The Stage)

Sara was 45, though she looked much older. Years of anorexia and heroin use had left her frail, exhausted and withdrawn. She had taken part in many treatments like medication, group programs, and psychotherapy. Each offered pieces of support but never a lasting sense of stability. During her first chair exercise, strong emotions surfaced. Sitting in the child chair, she was overwhelmed by feelings of worthlessness and fear. When she moved to the adult chair, she noticed how weak that part of her was: uncertain, quiet, almost absent. But less fearful. The child's mistrust of the adult was striking, and it reflected her history of being repeatedly let down. Yet the exercise gave her something new; a structure where her adult mode could begin to respond to her child mode and trust could slowly form between them. With time and repetition, she started to notice when the frightened child was speaking and when the adult could answer. That awareness gradually changed her daily life. She ended contact with unsafe people, moved to a more stable environment, and began to eat more regularly. For the first time, she could sense that an adult part of her was present and capable. That stability made it possible to begin trauma therapy for her childhood abuse, work that until then had always felt out of reach. She started playing the violin in the way she never thought was possible.

New Endings for Old Stories: Schema Therapy and Imagery Rescripting

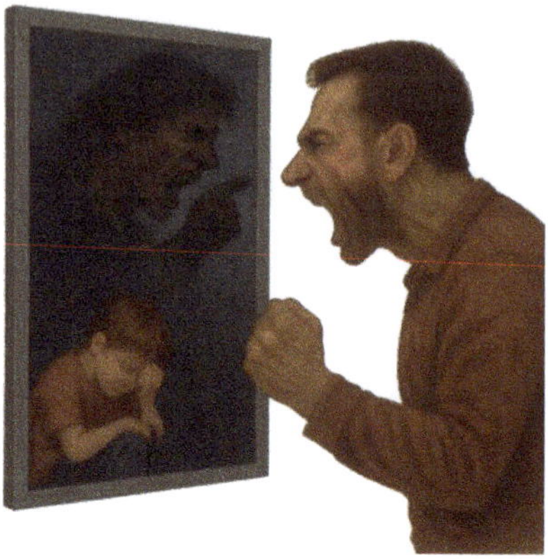

Imagery rescripting is a core technique in schema therapy, a full method in its own right. Here, I'll describe a simplified version that can be used safely in psychosomatic practice. Even in this form, it can reach emotional depths that words alone rarely touch.

The idea is straightforward but profound: the patient revisits painful childhood memories, but this time not as the helpless child, rather with the adult self present. The process begins with the patient imagining an old scene, a moment of fear, rejection, or loneliness. They step into it as the child, allowing the original emotions to appear. Once the image feels real, the second step begins: the adult self enters the scene. Now the child is no longer alone. Protection, care, or understanding become part of the memory. The goal is not to erase the past; the facts remain the same, but to give the nervous system a new experience: pain paired with safety. Sometimes the adult self cannot yet provide that protection. The patient may hesitate, freeze, or feel too weak. In such cases, the therapist can temporarily step into the image, standing beside the adult self and modeling how to protect and comfort the child. Over time, the patient takes over this role. The adult mode strengthens and the inner child learns what safety feels like, often for the first time.

Imagery rescripting changes the emotional meaning of a memory. For psychosomatic patients, this often reduces chronic bodily symptoms because the nervous system no longer reacts as if the trauma were still happening. The same method can be used for recurring nightmares: instead of reliving the same frightening scenes, patients rescript them. They bring in their adult self, or in early stages, the therapist's support. With practice, even nightmares lose their grip.

Safety always comes first. If anxiety rises too high, the exercise is paused, grounding is re-established, and only then does the work continue. The pace must always match the patient's capacity. The chair technique and imagery rescripting often complement each other. The chair exercise helps patients distinguish between child and adult modes. When progress stalls, imagery rescripting adds what's missing: the experience of protection. Together, they build self-trust and open the way toward even deeper trauma therapy. Try this method only if you have training in cognitive-behavioral methods. Otherwise, refer a patient to a specialist.

Case: Sara, The Thin Woman (Part II: Visiting Old "Friends")

After gaining stability with the chair technique, she was ready for imagery work. In one session, she pictured herself as an 8-year-old girl sitting at the family table. Her parents were cold, critical, and distant. As the child, she felt small and terrified, because she knew the beatings from her father were about to start. When she tried to bring in her adult self, she couldn't. The protective voice she needed was missing. At that point, the therapist entered the image, not as a rescuer but as support for Sara's adult self, standing beside her as she faced her parents. With that presence behind her, Sara could finally protect the child. She confronted the father for hurting the child and the mother for not stopping it. For the first time, her younger self was not abandoned. The effect carried into her life. She started to take care of her physical health, organizing different doctor appointments and trusting that she can be helped with the consequences of anorexia and heroin use. The chair work had helped her hear the child's voice; imagery rescripting helped her protect it. Together, these methods formed a bridge from insight to emotional repair. She started building the orchestra.

Calming the Mind, Protecting the Body: Meditation and Mindfulness

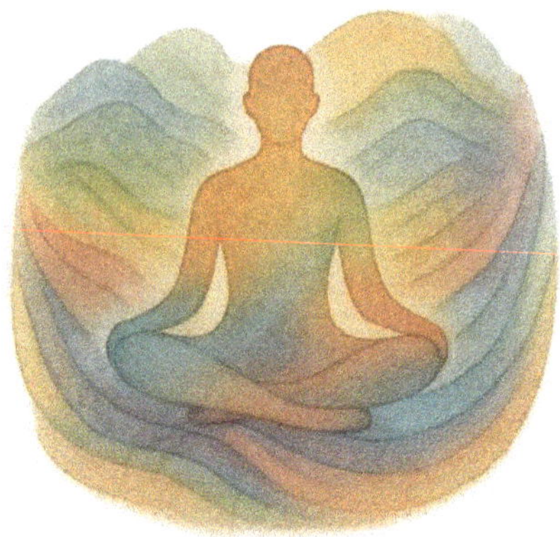

Meditation and mindfulness are not just relaxation tools; they are evidence-based methods that directly influence both mind and body. Research shows they help regulate stress responses, reduce symptom intensity, and, in some studies, are even associated with longer telomeres, a biological marker of slower cellular aging. It's not a cure or a guarantee of full recovery, but it shows how deeply such practices can affect health when done consistently.

The field of mindfulness-based interventions is vast, from *Mindfulness-Based Stress Reduction* and *Mindfulness-Based Cognitive Therapy,* to compassion-focused and trauma-sensitive approaches, but even basic techniques can be meaningful when introduced with care. *Breath awareness:* focusing attention on the inhale and exhale and gently returning to the breath whenever the mind drifts. *Body scan:* moving awareness slowly through the body, noticing sensations such as tension or pain without judgment or resistance. The body scan described in Chapter 2 focused on observing and shifting symptoms as a diagnostic tool; here, its purpose is to cultivate inner peace. *Observing thoughts:* watching thoughts as passing clouds rather than facts that demand reaction. *Self-compassion meditation:* placing a hand on the chest and silently repeating, *"May I be safe. May I be calm. May I be kind."* This act softens shame and activates the brain's soothing systems.

With regular practice, many patients notice that symptoms become less intense, stress reactions settle more quickly, and the connection between body and mind grows steadier. For some patients, it becomes a daily anchor; for others, an occasional experiment. Both are valid. The message is simple: mindfulness is one option; evidence-based, accessible, and safe. Mindfulness can also be practiced in movement and daily life, through a slow walk, a moment of listening or the rhythm of cooking, for those who find stillness uncomfortable. Even fifteen minutes a day can shift how the nervous system responds. Whether a patient chooses to use it or not is entirely up to them.

Your Perspective, Your Practice

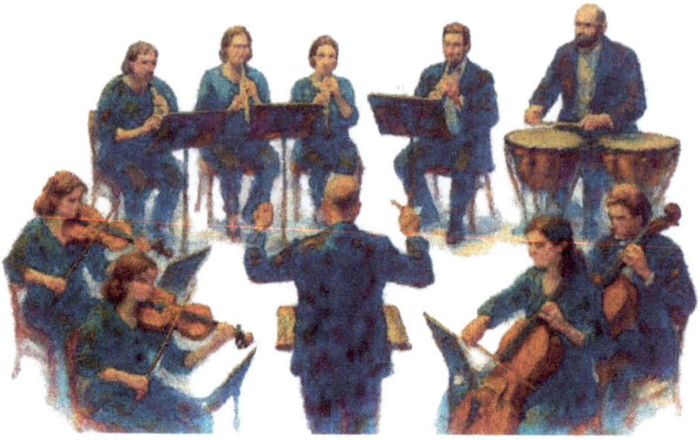

Psychosomatic work isn't about knowing every technique. It's about how you use yourself in the room. The tools matter, but your stance matters more. Start where the patient is. Stability comes before insight. Medication, structure and rest often do more in the beginning than interpretation. External stability matters just as much; housing, safety, and finances are part of calming the system before deeper work can begin. When the system calms, thinking can start again. Follow the symptom, but don't chase it.

The child part needs safety, warmth, and regulation. But with the adult mode, the approach changes. Here you can be clear, even firm. The adult mode often hides behind rationalization or avoidance; it needs structure and accountability. Setting limits firmly, without irritation or shame, helps the patient feel that someone is guiding the process. When done calmly, this firmness is containment and many patients experience it as genuine care.

In this field, rescue is a temptation. You see suffering and want to help. But containment works better than fixing. Patients learn from your calm more than from your advice. And don't forget your own body. Notice when you hold your breath, tense your shoulders, or feel heavy after sessions. These moments are not distractions but information. They reveal what the patient's world feels like from the inside and remind you where your own limits lie. You may know this as countertransference, not a theory but a lived form of empathy, a quiet response to another person's pain that passes through your body before it reaches the mind. For therapists who tend to suppress their own reactions, this awareness can be quietly transformative. Those signals are messages too. They show what kind of emotional climate you're working in and when you need to step out of it.

Progress in psychosomatic therapy is quiet. Symptoms fade like background noise. Patients often miss the moment when something shifts; you might see it first. Often the body shows progress before the mind can name it: a breath that deepens, a voice that steadies, a shoulder that finally drops. You can see it in posture, voice, or the way they say *"I think I can handle this."* Mark those moments. It helps both of you see that change is real. In most cases, patients start to talk and act like adults.

Stay patient, stay adult. The methods will follow naturally. Listen to the piece your patient is composing.

CHAPTER FOUR

The ISTDP Method

How To Approach Chapter Four

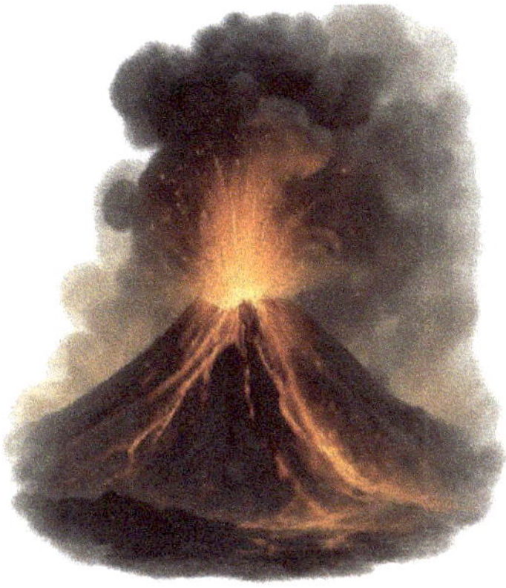

Think of a volcano before it erupts. Deep underground, pressure builds slowly, invisible to the eye. The mountain swells, the ground trembles, and for a long time everything stays contained. Then the moment comes: molten rock bursts through, smoke and fire fill the air, and the release is unstoppable. Afterwards, the air clears, the pressure is gone and something remarkable begins. Over time, the ash and lava break down, mixing with organic matter. What was once destructive can be some of the most fertile soil on earth: rich, alive, capable of supporting new growth.

That is what it can feel like in therapy when repressed emotion finally breaks through. Anger, sadness, impulses, and then suddenly a relief. The body softens, symptoms ease, and sometimes both patient and therapist even laugh. These moments remind us that emotions are not abstract forces. They live in the body. When blocked for too long, they press inward, generating pain and exhaustion until they are finally allowed to move again. And just like volcanic soil, once the eruption in therapy has passed, the inner ground grows fertile again. A place where resilience, connection and new patterns can grow.

Some methods even work directly with this process. Intensive Short-Term Dynamic Psychotherapy (ISTDP) is one of them. It targets the unconscious emotional pressures that create psychosomatic symptoms like chest tightness, headaches, abdominal pain and fatigue. Rather than staying stuck in endless investigation, ISTDP helps patients face, feel, and release the emotions that keep the body tense. ISTDP is a demanding method that requires advanced training and supervision, but its principles can enrich any clinician's work. Noticing how anxiety shows in the body, recognizing when defences block emotion, and inviting the patient to feel rather than explain. These are skills every therapist can use. Recent studies confirm what many clinicians observe: when the emotional core is reached, psychosomatic symptoms often ease. The body calms once it no longer has to carry what has finally been allowed to come to the surface.

This chapter takes you into that eruption: through fire, ash and finally the quiet ground where new life begins.

Three Forces at Play: The Triangle of Conflict

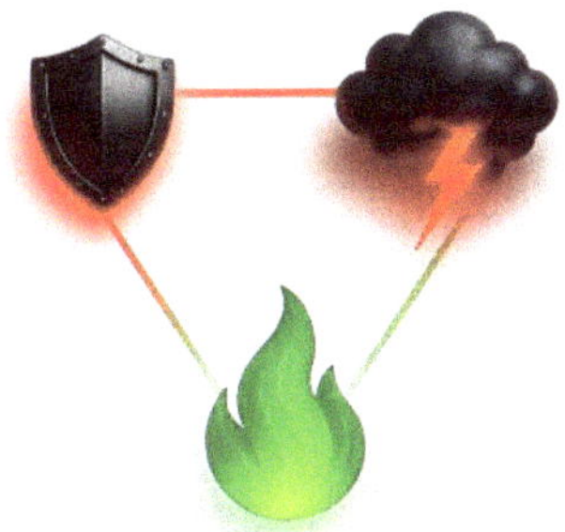

In Intensive Short-Term Dynamic Psychotherapy (ISTDP), the triangle of conflict offers a clear and practical way to understand what drives psychosomatic symptoms. At its three corners lie defences, anxiety, and feelings. The goal of therapy is to help patients move away from the red corners, defence and anxiety, toward the green corner where genuine feeling can finally emerge and integrate.

Defences are the first barrier. They can sound reasonable, even adaptive, but they distance a person from their emotional truth. Instead of sadness, a patient might joke. Instead of anger, they might intellectualize. Others insist they feel *"nothing at all."* These are not lies, but they are survival strategies, built long ago to manage what once felt unbearable. Defences take shape within relationships and social environments, not only within individual psychology; they once protected a person in the context they lived in, even if they now cause harm. In therapy, naming them without judgment helps loosen their grip. The aim is not to remove defences, but to make them flexible enough for feeling to pass through.

When emotions begin to push against those defences, **anxiety** rises. It is the body's way of signaling that something emotional has been activated, even if the mind has not caught up yet. Anxiety speaks in physical language: shallow breath, tight chest, clenched stomach, or pressure in the head. These are not emotions but physiological stress reactions. Over time, the brain can confuse the two, pairing emotion with bodily distress: anger equals migraine, sadness equals nausea. The person learns, without realizing it, that emotion is dangerous.

Beyond anxiety lies the third corner, **feeling**. It's the green zone of authentic experience. When emotions are felt directly, the body and mind move together. Sadness brings tears, anger brings heat, guilt softens into responsibility. And when this is expressed, the body relaxes. That is the natural completion of an emotional cycle.

Distinguishing between anxiety and emotion is crucial. Anxiety seems to follow anatomy, so you can witness stomach cramps, pounding headaches, shallow breathing, chest pressure... If you're good at anatomy, you can even know which neural pathway or plexus may be involved. Intense emotions are different. They spread through the body, hard to follow anatomically. By carefully observing both bodily responses and verbal descriptions, we can begin to tell them apart. And when the true feeling is reached, it almost always brings what was missing all along: a relief. Anxiety doesn't seem to bring relief.

Case: Michael and the Migraine

Michael, 38, suffered from recurrent migraines. All neurological tests were normal, yet the pain returned again and again, especially after tense interactions with his boss. Exploration revealed the triangle at work. Michael felt anger, but he never expressed it; he smiled, stayed polite and pushed it down. That was his defence. The emotion did not disappear; it moved into his body. His shoulders tightened, his jaw locked and soon the migraine came. This was the anxiety corner in action. In therapy, we mapped the triangle together: anger, anxiety, defence. Slowly, Michael allowed himself to feel the anger directly, to feel the heat in his chest and the urge to speak up. And something shifted. The migraine did not come. Relief followed because anger was finally allowed. Once the emotion moved through, the body no longer needed to carry it as pain. Even if it's only a small eruption of a vulcano, it's still an eruption.

Old Guards of the Mind: Defences

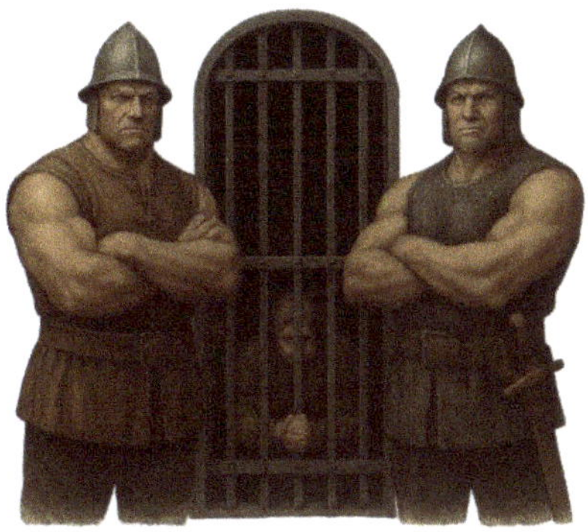

Defences are the ways we protect ourselves from anxiety and from emotions that once felt too dangerous to experience directly. They are not good or bad in themselves. At some point, every defence was a survival strategy. As children, we used them to keep relationships safe, to avoid punishment, or to shield ourselves from fear that felt unbearable. Many defences still make sense in ongoing unsafe environments, not just in childhood. Real change sometimes depends on improving those conditions, not only on gaining insight. In safer times, those same instincts could turn playful: a child might even manipulate a little to get a candy, harmless practice in how connection and need meet. But if that strategy becomes habitual, it can cause real harm in adult life: attempts to influence others may be read as deceitful or controlling, eroding trust and making close relationships harder to sustain. Over time, the emotion that was never spoken aloud stays trapped in the body and can feed symptoms rather than relieving them. Back then, those defenses helped us. But later in life these same strategies often come at a cost, because they block the very emotions that could now bring relief.

This is a complex area of psychology, with entire systems of classification. But in practice, we simplify it so that patients and therapists in training can recognize what is happening in real time. Some defenses are *mature,* like humor, or consciously putting a feeling aside for later. These can help people adapt and keep perspective. *Neurotic defenses,* such as overthinking (intellectualization), giving excuses (rationalization), or cutting emotion off from thought (isolation of affect), tend to keep a person in their head so the full emotion never lands. *Immature defenses,* like denial, projection, or acting out, are more disruptive. They remove awareness from the process entirely, leading to impulsive or confusing behaviors. And at the most fragile end are *malignant defenses,* such as splitting and severe distortion. These are often rooted in trauma and appear in people with more vulnerable personality organization.

When patients recognize their defenses without blame or shame, they begin to see both their purpose and their cost. By noticing when anxiety rises and defences take over, we can guide patients back toward the emotion underneath. The symptom does not vanish because the body is "fixed," but because the feeling has finally been felt.

Case: Dragan and the Chest Pain

Dragan, 42, came in with chronic chest pain. His heart had been checked repeatedly, no abnormalities, yet the pain always returned. When we explored stress, he began to talk about his father: a harsh, critical man who was never satisfied. As Dragan spoke, anger rose visibly; his jaw tightened, his shoulders stiffened, his hands trembled. But just as the emotion peaked, he smiled and said softly: "Oh well, it wasn't so bad. He just wanted the best for me." That smile was not joy. It was a defence, a quick rationalization to push the anger away. But the anger did not vanish; it moved into his body. His chest tightened, his breath shortened, and the familiar pain returned. We slowed down and tracked what happened. I pointed out the moment the pain appeared, exactly when he excused his father. Dragan paused, then quietly said, "Yes… I actually feel furious." As he stayed with the heat in his chest and the impulse to push back, the pain began to ease. He sighed deeply. The defence softened, and the real emotion, long frozen, finally had space. The volcano partially erupted.

Colors of Stress: Anxiety Pathways and the Traffic Light

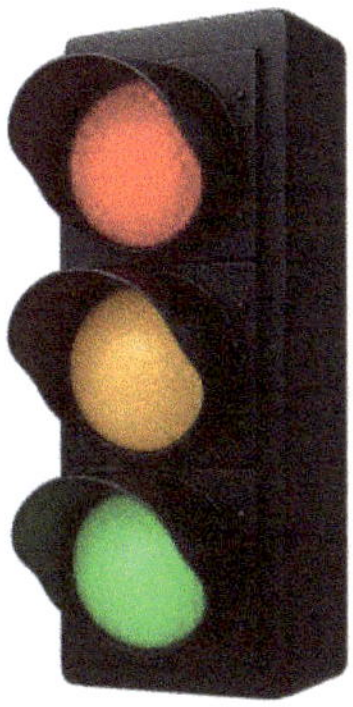

Anxiety in the body is not random. It follows distinct biological pathways. And when we learn to recognize them, we can separate stress reactions from genuine emotional experience.

In the **red zone**, bodily stress discharges directly into the brain. You suddenly see that a patient has problems with thinking and perception of the environment. If you're running from a bear, it's understandable that you might develop tunnel vision or even tinnitus, so you don't notice anything that could distract you from surviving. But in the therapists office, talking about emotions, it doesn't make sense. Unless… the alarm is oversensitive. The cognitive–perceptive system is overloaded, and in this state, no emotional processing is possible. The rule in red is always the same: stop, regulate and bring the system down before approaching emotion. Techniques such as grounding, slow breathing, or simply naming the overwhelm (*"I'm over my limit right now"*) help restore orientation.

In the **yellow zone**, bodily stress discharges into the autonomic nervous system. We are all familiar with those symptoms of anxiety, but the intensity of it when you talk about emotions makes a difference. The heart races, breathing becomes shallow, the stomach cramps and hands grow cold or sweaty. This is the tipping point between regulation and overload. Use the same rule as in red, if the symptoms are too strong: stop, regulate and bring the system down before approaching emotion.

In the **green zone**, activation flows through the motor system. At this level emotion can safely move through the body. Muscles tense and it can be very unpleasant, but it's still the green zone. Here, therapy can deepen, and emotion can complete its natural cycle, often followed by a *spontaneous sigh* - the body's sign that regulation has occurred. When we regulate the symptoms from the red or yellow zone, we actually activate the green zone. All the techniques that involve voluntary muscles (including breathing techniques) are actually activating green zone to regulate anxiety. Also on the long run. This way you can explain to a patient why is regular physical exercise important for stress regulation.

The traffic light model translates complex psychophysiology into a tool that both therapist and patient can use. For clinicians, it is a roadmap: proceed in green, regulate in yellow, stop in red. For patients, it becomes a daily compass: recognize bodily stress symptoms, sort it on the traffic light, stop what you are doing as soon as you can and regulate it. Anxiety is not the enemy; it is information. When understood this way, it becomes a guide rather than a threat, pointing the way toward safety and self-regulation.

Case: Tamara and the Stomach Cramps

Tamara, 34, was describing tension with a coworker. The story itself seemed ordinary until she turned her attention to what she felt in that moment. Within seconds, her breathing stopped mid-sentence. Her eyes fixed on the floor, face pale, shoulders lifted high. She said she felt dizzy, as if the room was too bright. This was the ***red zone****. The stress signal had reached the cognitive–perceptive system, flooding her capacity to think or feel. The body had mistaken anger for physical danger. Emotional exploration stopped there. Continuing would only intensify the overload. The focus shifted entirely to regulation and psychoeducation. Together we observed what her body was doing, the shallow breath, the racing pulse, the narrowed awareness, and named it as a biological alarm, not a psychological failure. We practiced slow orientation: noticing the room, feeling the chair, lengthening the exhale. Gradually, her breathing found rhythm again. The dizziness eased. By the end of the session, we hadn't spoken further about the coworker. The work that day was to understand what the body had shown, that before emotion can be* *explored, safety must return. The lesson wasn't insight into anger, but recognition of the red zone itself: when the brain is defending, not feeling.*

The Spark Inside: Feelings and Impulses

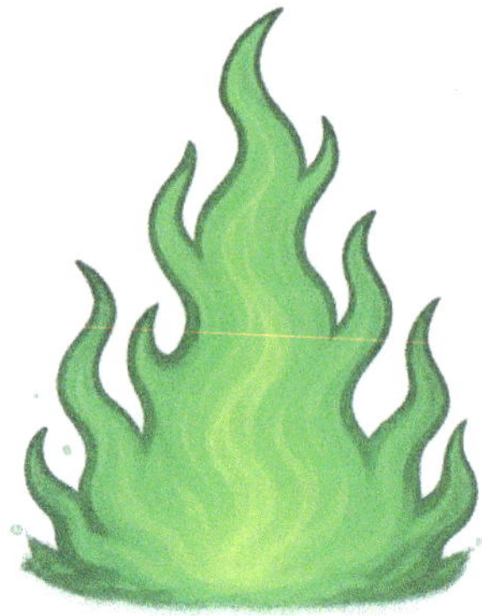

Every intense emotion carries an impulse. Love brings the impulse to come closer, to hold, to touch. Sadness carries the impulse to cry. Joy brings laughter, sometimes even tears. And anger carries the raw impulse to strike. These impulses are not conscious choices; they arise automatically from the nervous system, quick and unfiltered. They are part of how emotion moves through the body. We can't choose what we feel, only whether we face it or turn away. The feeling itself is there regardless. What we can shape is the reaction that follows, the impulse that rises with it.

Yet in working with anger, something else almost always appears right behind it: guilt. The moment the impulse to strike is felt, guilt often rushes in. As children, many of us learned that anger toward parents or caregivers was dangerous. To preserve the bond, anger was pushed down. This is the anger–impulse–guilt chain, one of the most common patterns in psychosomatic patients. Once patients learn that anger can be felt safely, they often regain both emotional freedom and physical vitality. Love and anger are not opposites. If a patient can be angry at someone close without fearing to lose them, that relationship is strong. If they cannot, then perhaps they need to see it more realistically, especially when it comes to family relationships in adult life.

In therapy, this chain can often be seen directly in the body: a tightening posture, clenched hands, then a sudden slump or tears. Sometimes it can even be felt in the therapist's own body. This is transference and countertransference at work, the shared field where the patient's inner conflict becomes visible. A trained therapist can feel a patient's defenses as irritation, impatience, or a sense of distance; the subtle *"they're getting on my nerves"* moment that signals resistance in the air. When anxiety rises in the patient, the therapist's body often joins in: a faster heartbeat, shallow breathing, a wish to soothe or rescue. And when genuine feeling finally emerges, something shifts in both; the therapist's shoulders drop, breath deepens, and a quiet relief spreads through the room. The system settles together. The therapist can *feel* the triangle of conflict and know where the process stands; the work continues until raw emotion finally comes to the surface.

Case: The Volcano of Helena

Helena was sixty-five and had lived much of her life under threat. She came to us after years of emergency-room visits for chest pain, dizziness, and abdominal distress; symptoms that always hinted at danger but never pointed to disease. Thirty years earlier, she had endured a decade of physical and psychological abuse from her partner, a man whose work was to help others heal. He eventually died of cancer; that was how she escaped. For a long time, Helena could not speak of it. Therapy, over time, gave her enough distance to look back without being engulfed. She "knew" she was angry. One day we decided to follow that knowledge into the body itself. When asked where she felt the anger, the first sensations came quickly: dizziness deepened, her stomach clenched, and her heart raced. We began as usual: naming and rating each symptom, mapping how the body responded. Then we stepped back for a moment, helping her think about what was happening so that reflection could soften fear. Then came a long sigh: my clue that her nervous system was beginning to regulate. Her breathing steadied, and the tension shifted into her shoulders and arms. The system seemed ready to mobilize instead of collapse. I invited her to stay with the anger toward the man who had hurt her. Again, symptoms surged; her arms went weak, as if energy drained away. I asked her what she felt toward ***me*** *right then. When she could sense trust and gratitude, her body released. The dizziness eased, her color returned. From that steadier ground, I invited her once more to feel anger; this time she could. A wave of heat rose through her torso into her face. Her arms moved with life once more. Helena spoke in a firm, trembling voice: "I am so angry at him." The rage had* *found its image, sharp and dangerous, yet held safely inside imagination. Guilt came quickly, cooling the surge. She stayed with both currents: the urge to strike and the shame that followed until they met and began to dissolve. Then she grew quiet. In her mind, something was laid to rest. Her muscles loosened, breath deepened, and the long-held tension gave way to tears. The impulse had found a voice. When she caught her breath, she looked up and said softly, "I don't know why, but my father came to mind." Something in the landscape had changed. The volcano that had rumbled underground for decades had finally erupted, not to destroy, but to release pressure that had kept her body in constant alarm. After the session, we focused on safety: grounding, hydration, slow breathing, and a plan for gentle days ahead. In the following weeks, Helena reported fewer emergency visits and a calmer body. The sessions that followed brought smaller aftershocks—more memories, more defences, but also a growing steadiness. The ground began to turn fertile again, quiet and alive beneath her feet.*

Touching the Core: Breakthrough to the Unconscious

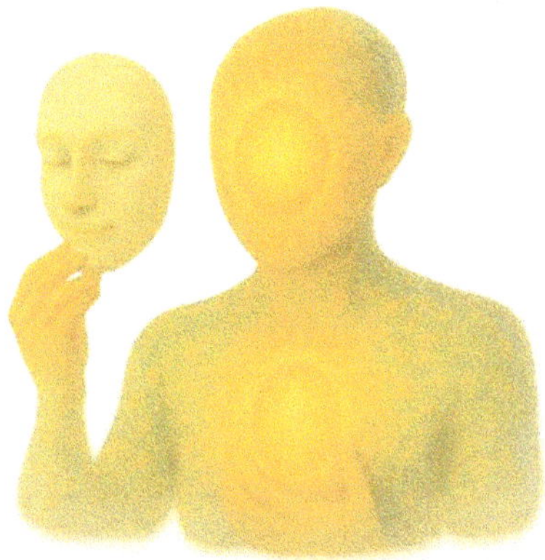

In Intensive Short-Term Dynamic Psychotherapy (ISTDP), one of the central goals is a breakthrough to the unconscious: a moment when emotion, memory, and body reconnect. It's not just remembering; it's feeling something deeply and knowing where it comes from. Anger toward a boss today suddenly resonates with the anger once forbidden toward a parent. Grief after a present loss awakens the grief of a childhood without comfort or protection. This linking of past and present is not random. It is guided by the therapeutic alliance, the trust that allows a patient to face what was once unbearable. In ISTDP, that inner readiness is called the unconscious therapeutic alliance (UTA): an instinct in the patient that wants truth to surface and senses safety in the therapist. Breakthroughs cannot be forced. They emerge when defenses soften and the nervous system feels secure enough to let feeling flow.

When a breakthrough occurs, the shift is unmistakable. The body releases years of tension, breathing deepens, and emotion floods through. Vital signs often settle, color returns, muscle tone softens. What once felt stuck begins to move. Symptoms that seemed permanent may ease or disappear, as if the nervous system finally resets its rhythm. It is like volcanic soil. The eruption itself may have been violent long ago, but what follows is ground made fertile. A breakthrough clears the hardened crust of old defenses and leaves behind inner soil where resilience, strength, and freedom can take root. Practically, that means patients often continue to develop long after the short, intensive therapy has ended, they live differently, breathe differently, and relate differently.

A breakthrough to the unconscious is not just a clinical event; it is the body reorganizing around a truth that can finally be felt. Guided by safety and trust, patients discover that what once had to be hidden can now be faced without collapse. Not every session reaches this depth, and not every patient is ready. But when it happens, the transformation is palpable: beneath anxiety and defenses, there is always life waiting to move, to feel, to be released.

Case: Daniel and the Breakthrough

Daniel, forty-one, came to therapy with severe headaches and chronic muscle tension. In one session, he described an argument with a close friend. His jaw tightened, fists curled and he admitted feeling an impulse to punch, to lash out physically. For the first time, he let himself imagine it fully: the movement, the heat, the force. Almost instantly, guilt followed. His shoulders slumped, his eyes dropped, and the headache flared right there in the room. We stayed with it. He noticed the anger again, then the guilt, then the heaviness that sat behind both. As he traced it deeper, the image of his parents surfaced. The rage he felt toward his friend was the same rage he had carried since childhood, toward a father who had humiliated and belittled him. Beneath it lay another, quieter current: the anger toward his mother for not protecting him, long suppressed and wrapped in loyalty. When he mentioned her, he paused for a moment, his eyes unfocused, then quickly shifted back to his father. It was the father who still filled the room; his presence lived on in the patient's body, in every flash of tension and defiance. The connection clicked into place: present and past joined in one embodied feeling. When that realization came, his whole body changed. His breathing slowed, his face softened, and for the first time he said quietly, "It wasn't just my friend. I've been angry at my father all my life." Tears followed. The tension in his neck released, the headache eased. In the sessions that followed, Daniel's headaches grew less frequent. He described a new steadiness, a sense that his body no longer needed to shout for him to listen. Three months later, the change was unmistakable. His body moved more freely, sleep deepened, appetite returned, and laughter showed up in moments that used to tighten him. The ground beneath his life had become very fertile. Still, a small worry lingered in me: the silence around his mother. It remained a blind spot, a place he hadn't yet approached. But for now, the movement was good, and I chose to trust it. He can return at any time for another short, intensive block of therapy if life brings the next layer to the surface

Learning To Ride a Bike: Acting Fast with ISTDP

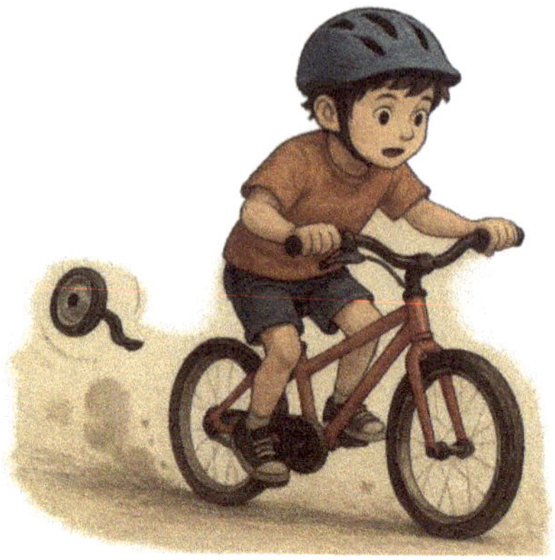

ISTDP isn't easy to do. It asks for intensive training, regular supervision, and a steady therapeutic frame. What you can do right away is psychoeducation: teach the triangle of conflict, use the traffic-light model for anxiety, and help patients spot their own defences. These ideas are safe, clear, and already useful.

A full ISTDP session is different. In a specialist practice, the first session can last up to three hours. A hallmark is speed with precision. Done well, this bypasses the usual avoidance. The shift can feel sudden: before the machinery locks down, the buried emotion rises and a breakthrough occurs. This is not recklessness. It's calibrated pressure in small doses, paired with instant monitoring of yellow and red, and swift regulation whenever needed. The speed protects the work; it does not overwhelm the patient. Because the method is demanding, patients give informed, written consent. Sessions are often video-recorded for supervision. Reviewing the video shows what eyes and ears miss: micro-defences, the exact moment a sigh signals regulation, or the clenching of the hands.

A word of caution. It is wise to begin learning this method; it is unwise to attempt its forceful manoeuvres without proper training and supervision. Techniques involving sustained pressure, moment-to-moment blocking of complex defences, or safely working with violent impulses require a solid skill base, a clear red, yellow, and green map, and sometimes live supervision. Safe first steps: educate, recognise patterns, build presence, and practise anxiety regulation. The deeper, faster interventions belong to formal training and careful mentoring.

At its best, intensive therapy is like teaching someone to ride a bike. In the beginning, therapist and patient move together, both emotionally invested in finding balance. The therapist steadies the handlebars, guides the rhythm, and helps the patient stay upright through the early uncertainty. As confidence grows, the therapist begins to let go. Regulation becomes internal, and the patient starts to feel their own strength. The safety of the therapist's presence gives way to something deeper: trust in one's own capacity to move forward. Letting go is both tender and necessary. The therapist steps back, and the patient rides on, unsteady for a moment, then free, carried by their own momentum.

Your Perspective, Your Practice

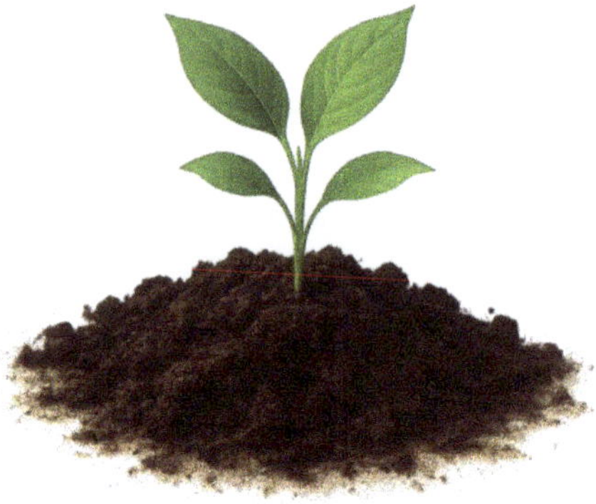

Wherever you stand in the healthcare system, you already have tools to make a difference.

If you work in *general medicine,* you can transform a patient's experience simply by naming what happens in the body. Explain the triangle of conflict, validate that symptoms are real, and show how stress travels through the nervous system.

If you are a *specialist* who meets patients after years of referrals and inconclusive tests, you have the chance to open the door to psychosomatic therapies such as ISTDP. These approaches can save years of unnecessary investigation and bring genuine relief. Research consistently shows that when you explain the body–mind connection clearly and with empathy, patients' distress decreases and healthcare use declines.

If you are a *psychotherapist*, you can apply these principles directly. Ask about feeling, notice defences, and support patients as they regulate anxiety. Rooted in broader psychodynamic traditions, ISTDP shares the same aim: to bring unconscious emotion into awareness, but it does so with greater precision and immediacy through direct focus on the body's response.

If you are a *nurse* or another frontline clinician, you often see the effects of emotional tension first. Your steady presence between sessions, your ability to notice small shifts in breath, posture, or tone, and your quiet reassurance during moments of distress make integration possible.

If you are a *social worker*, you extend this work beyond the therapy room. By helping patients build safer environments, strengthen families, and reconnect with community, you translate emotional healing into daily life. Psychosomatic recovery depends not only on inner change but also on outer conditions that support it.

Each encounter, each moment of real contact, is like tending volcanic ground. The work is to stay present through the eruption, and then to help what follows take root. That is where healing becomes fertile.

CHAPTER FIVE

Clinical Thinking For Complex Presentations

How To Approach Chapter Five

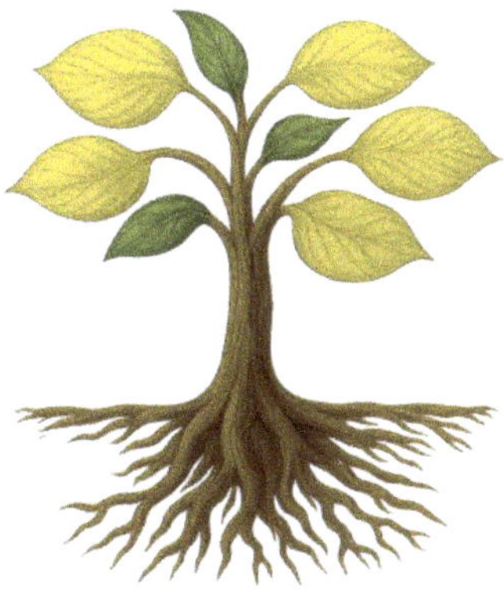

When patients come with chronic body pain, fatigue, migraines, insomnia, or gut distress, the picture looks scattered, a handful of unrelated problems. At the top are the visible **leaves**: the symptoms patients describe. The **trunk** holds their story: how relationships, safety, and early stress shaped the ways they learned to cope. Beneath lie the **roots**: genetics, wiring, and resilience. Some roots are sturdy, others tangled, but they can still be tended. Below them is the **soil**, the unseen layer of family history and social world. When someone finally sees your whole tree, not just the leaves, something shifts. The body stops defending and begins to breathe.

Before we move to the cases, where we will craft trees together, we need tools for that craft. Working with a tree is like gardening: it requires patience, timing, and care. You do not force growth; you create the conditions for it. The gardener learns when to water, when to prune, and when to wait. The same applies in clinical work. To work with the tree, we can use three tools. *The Listening Mind* stays steady in confusion, catching meaning beneath words. *The Skilled Hand* turns insight into timing, knowing when to ask, when to pause, when to act. *The Steady Heart* builds trust, the physiology of safety where healing takes root. These three tools may sound abstract, but the next sections will bring them to life through real cases, where each finds its form in practice.

Understanding a tree takes time. It keeps changing as trust deepens and new layers appear. But it is better to spend (for example) two years restoring what can truly change, the body's balance, the mind's flexibility, the safety of connection, than twenty circling the same confusion. Still, the idea of spending two years on one restoration may sound idealistic in a system where maybe ten sessions are all that is allowed. That tension matters too.

In practice, trees do not always grow back. Some remain marked by the storms they endured. Recognizing that, without losing hope, gives our work its quiet authority. Each tree is shaped by weather beyond its control. Our task is not to prune away the leaves too soon, but to understand how they grew, and to help balance return, in whatever form it can. Without that wider view, the tree risks looking solitary, when in truth it stands within a forest shaped by care systems, social forces, and the unequal climates we all live in.

The Listening Mind: The Compass of Clinical Thinking

When a patient begins to talk, the room fills fast. Symptoms, test results, half-formed fears, stories that shift mid-sentence. Some are clear, some tangled. *The Listening Mind* steadies you in that flood. It listens and thinks at the same time, aware that every sentence might hold meaning. Beneath the story, something deeper is trying to be heard. It's like tuning a radio, waiting for the faint signal to cut through static.

You hold the Compass Questions quietly in mind: *Why now? Why this? Why here?* And sometimes, *Why does this get under my skin?* They belong to psychodynamic traditions: keep you oriented, stop you from chasing detail, and point you back to what matters. Countertransference joins the compass as a clue. When irritation or sympathy rises, you ask: *Why this feeling in me?* Patients rarely arrive with the whole story. Shame, habit, or pain can disguise the core message. So you listen differently. When a word lands heavier than others, when a pause breaks rhythm, when emotion flickers... you mark it. Those are your coordinates. As you hold the compass, the outline of the patient's tree begins to form. When the hinge sentence finally comes, the one that shifts the whole picture, you feel it. The noise thins, direction returns. For the patient, that hinge can bring relief, fear, or exposure, as if something long buried has just been named.

Not every story ends in clarity. Sometimes the signal never fully clears, and that is part of the work too. The following cases show how this tool works in practice. If you can find even a few such moments in your own work, it is already a success.

Case: Eric, the patient who "uses the system"

Eric, thirty-three, carries a folder thick with normal test results, chest tightness, dizziness, stomach pain. On paper, he looks like someone using the system without reason. That's when you hold your compass and ask quietly: Why does he keep coming back? Why do I feel impatient? He talks and talks, headaches, job stress, sleeplessness, tram rides. It's all noise until one line lands: "Nights are the worst. The place is too quiet." That's your hinge. Why nights? He circles around it, says he leaves the TV on, can't stand silence. Then another sentence slips out: "I try not to think about... the old stuff." Now you're close. Why avoid the old stuff? What old stuff? Then the picture forms: a violent father, nights when silence meant danger. The body learned vigilance as survival, and decades later it still stands guard. Eric isn't abusing the system; he's searching for safety. His symptoms are his body's language for 'still not safe'. The next step isn't another test; it's one clinician he can trust, a calmer evening routine, and trauma-focused therapy.

Case: Nina, the woman who is always tired

Nina, forty, apologizes as she sits down. Blood work fine, scans clean. Nothing explains her exhaustion. You hold the compass: Why so tired? What am I feeling as she talks? She describes work, emails, deadlines, a boss who never sleeps. Stress, yes, but not enough. You wait. Then she says, "By the time I get home, I'm already bracing." There it is. Why bracing? She hesitates, then admits, "I never know which version of him I'll get." Now the map sharpens. Her partner drinks. She hides it, manages everything, constantly on alert. Her body isn't weak; it's overloaded. Fatigue is the biology of vigilance. She's not here for another test; she's here because the life she's maintaining is unsustainable. What helps isn't a supplement. It's understanding stress biology, building boundaries, and creating small, protected spaces for recovery.

Case: Marko, the back pain that isn't just back pain

Marko, fifty-two, asks for stronger painkillers. His MRI shows wear and tear, nothing dramatic. Heavy job, stiff mornings, the usual story. Yet the pain never improves. You keep the compass steady: Why this pain, in this way? Why do I feel a heaviness as he speaks? He talks about failed exercises and sleepless nights, until a hinge appears: "Rest isn't an option." That catches you. Why not? More details, and then the sentence that unlocks the case: "My mother can't stand. I lift her." Now the pattern opens. He is the only caregiver, lifting her in and out of bed every day. His pain is real, and so is his load. The problem isn't just his spine; it's the structure of his life. The plan shifts: home support, safe-transfer training, physiotherapy. Pain eases because the world around it does.

The Skilled Hand: The Craft of Clinical Action

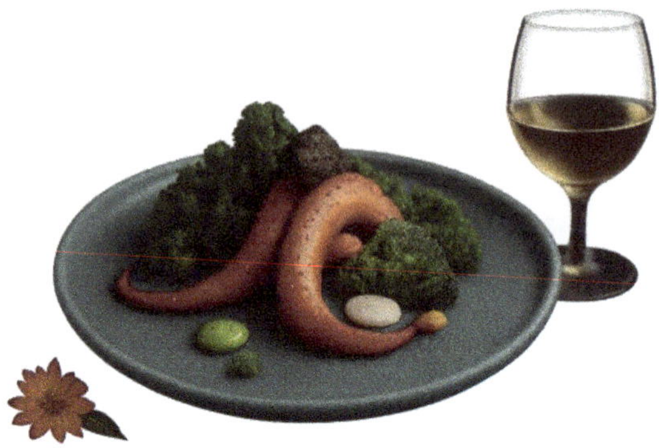

Think of a fine-dining kitchen, just for comparison. The pantry is not magic: the same ingredients, the same tools. The difference is the craft, what you prepare first, what you pair, when you add heat, and when you let something rest. Clinical thinking in psychosomatic care works the same way. The ingredients are right there: symptoms, history, examination, and context. The result depends on how you notice, what you connect, and when you act or wait.

In complex cases, this way of working keeps you from drowning in detail. It gives you a frame so fragments start speaking to each other. Not harder work, but sharper work. Which question matters now? Which test would actually change the plan? When is it wiser to pause and let the body show its next move? Sometimes you wait and let the picture develop. That time is not empty; it is how clarity arrives without burning you or the patient out. Even with experience, there are moments when you still hesitate, unsure which element to touch first. That pause is not weakness; it is respect for complexity. When a patient meets a clinician who works this way, they often feel it before they understand it. The room becomes calmer, the questions slower, and for the first time the story begins to make sense.

You are not a one-person kitchen. Specialists, laboratories, and imaging all run their stations. And the patient, too, brings their own ingredients: history, effort, and will. Your role is to balance what everyone contributes and turn it into one coherent meal of care. Job title does not guarantee that view; attention does. And sometimes you are the only one in the room who can connect the dots, whatever your role in health care. *The Skilled Hand* is technical, but also responsive. It senses when the patient's system is ready for challenge and when it needs rest. It takes what the *Listening Mind* has found, set the order of operations, choose when to touch and when to wait, and shape a plan that holds together.

We will stay inside that process. Not theory first, but messy reality: too many complaints, stories that do not match, and signals that pull against each other. Step by step, you will watch clinical craft turn noise into pattern and fragments into a whole you can act on, until the ingredients of daily practice come together like a finished dish, balanced, nourishing, and clear.

The Steady Heart: The Therapeutic Alliance

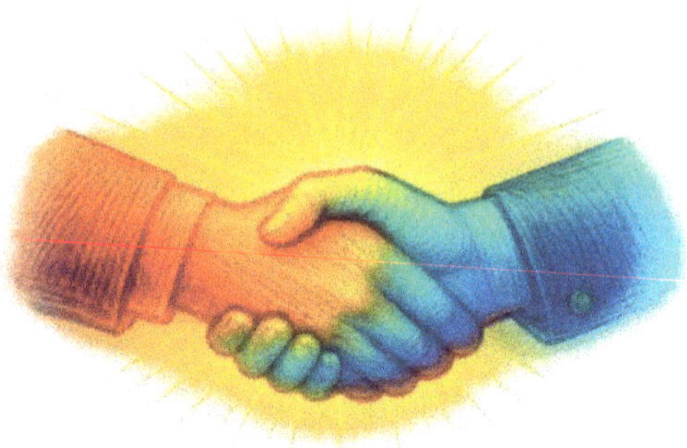

You can listen well and act precisely, yet nothing moves without trust. The tree cannot grow in cold air. What opens patients is not your questions or your plan, but your presence, the steady field that tells their body it is safe enough to shift.

The therapeutic alliance is not a matter of manners. It is the ground all technique grows from. The body feels safety before the mind does. That is why pain can ease after a few calm breaths, not only from oxygen or vagal tone but because the patient feels you breathing with them. Regulation is shared. The body tests the air, finds it steady, and lowers its guard. Yet resonance is not always calm. Sometimes your own system joins the distress before balance returns. That too belongs to the work.

Safety does not always come. Trust can resist growth, especially after betrayal or trauma. You keep offering steadiness without demand, knowing that even the absence of trust tells a story worth hearing. When safety begins to form, the patient feels it first in the body, in the moment they stop performing and simply exist. In that quiet, the deeper alliance begins. Patients connect dots on their own, remember what was missing, and link symptoms with feeling. They give you more material for the tree, clearer leaves, visible roots, a trunk that holds. Without that ground, even the best tools are like metal dropped on frozen soil: sharp but useless.

Co-regulation is not a metaphor. It can be measured. Heart rate, breathing, and tone shift together when safety returns, as biofeedback studies show. When trust enters the room, physiology follows and what once seemed fixed starts to move.

Case: The Puzzle of Pain

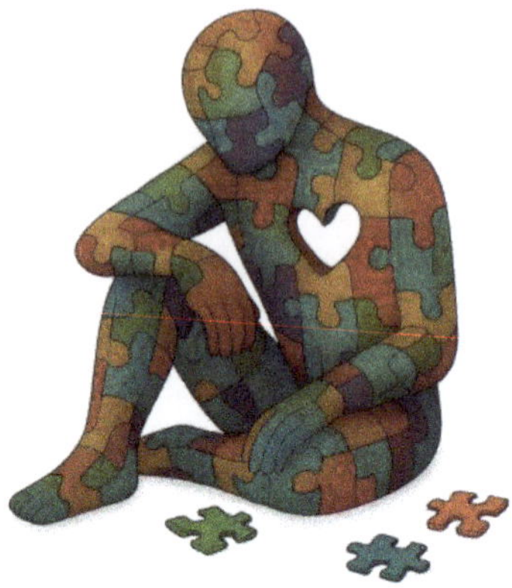

Oliver is thirty-two. He comes because his back will not stop hurting. That is the leaf that finally brings him in. As we talk, other leaves appear: fatigue that clings, stomach cramps that strike without reason, headaches that tighten by afternoon, nights broken by restless sleep. The work-up is textbook thorough: MRI, labs, neurological exam, all normal. I start with the usual psychosomatic groundwork: psychoeducation, pacing, relaxation, sleep hygiene. Within weeks, some leaves fade, headaches ease, the stomach quiets, sleep steadies. But the back pain stays, solid and unmoved. The reduction is fast but partial. We are far from done. I stay curious instead of frustrated. Pain that resists quick wins usually points deeper. We keep treatment gentle and consistent, regulating before analyzing. The alliance forms here; steadiness matters more than answers.

Leaves: back pain, fatigue, stomach cramps, headache, insomnia.

The trunk parts do not come up right away. For weeks, Oliver stays polite, factual, focused on exercises. I sense more beneath but do not push. The therapeutic relationship is the real beginning; without it, information is noise. Only later, in small pieces, the story forms. School was chaos. He was *"lazy but smart,"* losing assignments, forgetting details, always behind. Teachers called him careless, not restless. My gut had twitched earlier, but I had not listened. Or maybe I was right to wait. The space between questions did the work. He tells me how he survived: overcorrecting, double-checking, working late, perfectionism as scaffolding. Then home tension, parents arguing, the air thick, him bracing. I feel the same tightness across my own shoulders as he speaks. I notice my countertransference; his restlessness stirs my own. I let that discomfort guide me instead of defending against it. I invite small body-awareness experiments: unclench the jaw, let shoulders drop, follow one long exhale. His pain dips, briefly. I name what I see: *"You learned to brace early; your body still has not unlearned it."* The recognition lands deeper than any stretch.

Trunk: school chaos, disorganization, perfectionism, overcompensation, chronic bracing, parental conflict.

A few sessions later, he mentions a brother who cannot sit through dinner and a father who paces during TV shows. My mind tightens in focus, not as conclusion but as question. We complete a full developmental assessment: DIVA test, collateral history, and a conversation with his father. The pattern is clear, lifelong attention dysregulation, chronic overarousal, inherited restlessness. I hold both excitement and restraint, not rushing the label, listening for fit. I normalize: *"This does not erase who you are; it explains how your system runs."* ADHD (Attention-Deficit/Hyperactivity Disorder) is confirmed after thorough assessment. Medication begins, a stimulant carefully titrated. His back pain drops first with time, then fatigue. His energy steadies, concentration holds, the body's baseline tension quiets.

Roots: inherited attention problems, chronic hyperarousal, lifelong inattention, neurodevelopmental sensitivity.

Stories from family surface slowly. Grandparents displaced by war, a thread of endurance and anxiety running through generations. He lives alone, works long hours, shoulders quiet pressure to finally get it right. His body inherited vigilance as much as genes. I keep the historical lens open but light, context not destiny.

Soil: intergenerational stress, war displacement, anxiety lineage, perfectionist culture, social isolation.

We integrate structure around rest, realistic scheduling, and external cues. We also build concrete self-care routines: daily outdoor time, fixed meal rhythm, and short movement breaks that reconnect body and mind. Physiotherapy complements this process, teaching safe motion and postural release without reinforcing fear. The coordination between somatic and psychological work matters; the body learns best when mind and movement align. Alongside medication, we deepen the emotional process. Emotion-focused sessions help him notice early activation, regulate tension before it peaks, and name frustration or guilt without shame. Over months, Oliver's body loosens. The back pain still murmurs under stress, but its grip is weaker. For the first time in years, he says, *"I can sit without thinking about sitting."* I feel it too; our sessions breathe more easily. The turning point was naming the hidden root.

Research now links ADHD and chronic pain closely: shared mechanisms of hyperarousal, altered pain perception, and emotion dysregulation. Yet many of us overlook it. We do not think developmental when we see musculoskeletal, but often we should. My experience shows that emotion-focused therapies can complement ADHD treatment well. Research supports this: emotion dysregulation is a common and clinically relevant feature of ADHD, and interventions that address emotional processing improve overall functioning and reduce somatic complaints. Medication opens the window for emotional learning; therapy fills it with skill. Not every patient with ADHD reacts as well as Oliver, and not every pain hides ADHD. Still, it would be a shame to miss it when the match fits, when the missing piece is developmental, not mechanical. In such cases, recovery can be deep.

When symptoms don't follow the usual logic, pause and look again. What seems fixed can start to move when you listen from another angle. But what if ADHD is there, yet not alone? Let's turn to the next case.

Case: The Fire Below the Scar

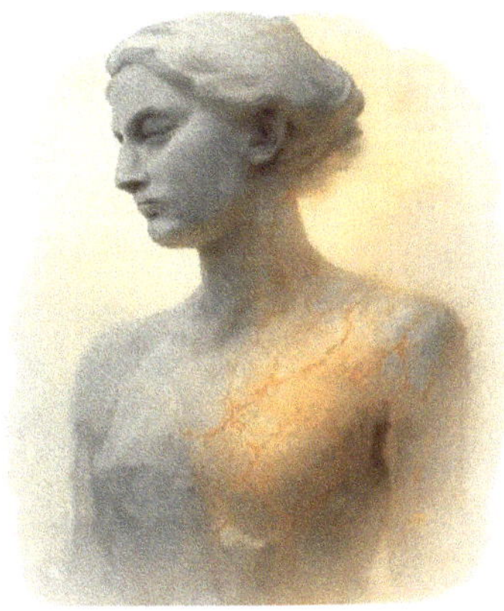

Sofia is twenty-eight when she first comes with irritable bowel symptoms: bloating, cramps, alternating diarrhea and constipation. That is the leaf that troubles her most. Soon, more leaves appear: increasing allergic reactions, and insomnia. She also suffers from recurrent depression, currently stabilized with medication. The work-up is thorough: colonoscopy, labs, allergy tests. All results return within normal limits, except for mild, nonspecific inflammation that explains little and offers no clear answer for her distress. Not alarming; also not enough to explain her suffering. The picture fits psychosomatic medicine, or better said, a biopsychosocial pattern, so treatment begins with psychoeducation, body-based regulation, and rhythm in daily life.

Leaves: IBS-like symptoms, allergies, recurrent depression, insomnia, mild nonspecific inflammation.

That's when you start noticing the trunk. Sofia grew up in a house without safety: neglect, abuse, unstable caregiving. The nervous system she carries was built in that weather. She commits fully to therapy and works hard. Over two years, progress is real: her gut stabilizes, sleep improves, and she completes a course of trauma therapy. Some leaves fall. But when you look again, the tree still feels incomplete. Something deeper keeps the system tense. Outside therapy, her life stays chaotic. Relationships swing between idealization and rejection. Anger comes fast, despair even faster. Therapists are adored, then abruptly cut off. Regulation and trauma work helped, but not the structure underneath. For a while it seemed the trauma work would be enough. But as symptoms returned, I began to wonder what still held the system so tightly. Tightening the transitions here, from trauma to the underlying traits, was essential both in therapy and in understanding her. Looking closer, another layer appeared. To survive, she clung to people, terrified of being left. Every small rupture felt like threat. By adolescence, emotional storms and impulsivity had hardened into an enduring pattern, a long-learned way of surviving that keeps hurting her now. This is what we clinically call *a borderline personality structure:* an inner system that still lives in the logic of threat and loss. Trauma therapy reached the past, but it lacked the stable frame she needed in the present; the work became too raw, too fast.

Trunk: early neglect, unstable caregiving, ongoing family stress, unstable attachment, fear of abandonment, emotional reactivity, impulsivity.

Beneath the developmental story lies a biological rhythm: distractibility, sensitivity to stimulation, subtle inner tension rather than visible hyperactivity. Traits on the ADD (Attention-Deficit Disorder) spectrum. Not a separate diagnosis here, but a temperament that keeps her system fast, easily flooded, and hard to calm. I wondered if this layer had been there all along, masked by the emotional turbulence above it.

Roots: ADD-spectrum traits, low threshold for autonomic arousal, inherited temperament.

Her mother struggled with depression and unstable relationships; her grandmother with unspoken trauma. The chemistry of stress was in the ground long before Sofia was born.

Soil: maternal instability, depression, intergenerational trauma.

Now the picture sharpens. Trauma is part of it, but not the whole frame. Beneath the symptoms lies a borderline personality structure built from developmental stress and inherited vulnerability. Early therapy eased the surface but not the deeper system that kept creating new crises. Diagnosis takes time. Most of the time you don't see a personality disorder at first glance. Patients also rarely show everything: the self-harm, the fights, the collapses. You sense it before you name it; the story never quite fits. And remember, nobody comes if everything is fine.

For Sofia, the turn came with Dialectical Behavior Therapy with an experienced psychotherapist, a structured frame strong enough to hold her storms. Slowly, her relationships steadied. For the first time, she described calm as something she could feel: her body loose, her chest open, the room suddenly wide and quiet. Meanwhile, medical follow-up continued in parallel with regular check-ins, and reassurance that nothing physical was missed. At the same time, her outer world remained fragile. Work was unstable, her finances tight, family contact strained. These pressures kept feeding the system, reminding us that no therapy stands apart from life itself.

Sofia's case shows why psychosomatic medicine demands patience and repeated depth checks. You don't stop at trauma; you follow the tree downward, leaves, trunk, roots, soil, until the whole structure comes into view. Here, early regulation and trauma therapy helped symptoms but left the deeper system untouched. The hidden pattern, borderline personality structure with ADD-like traits, explained why progress stalled. These two temperaments amplify each other: ADD fuels distractibility and inner tension; the personality structure magnifies emotional storms and attachment instability. The result is a body that never truly stands down. Not every chronic case hides such a structure. But when progress stops making sense, it's time to look again at the tree. Sometimes what seems like resistance is simply something still unseen. We shouldn't label everything with a diagnosis, but if you avoid naming what's there and confronting it, patients can circle for years in therapy.

Once the full pattern is recognized, therapy stops chasing symptoms and starts changing the system itself. But what if you cannot change it? What if the tree is already formed, its shape set by time and biology? Let's look at the next case.

Case: Anatomy of Suffering

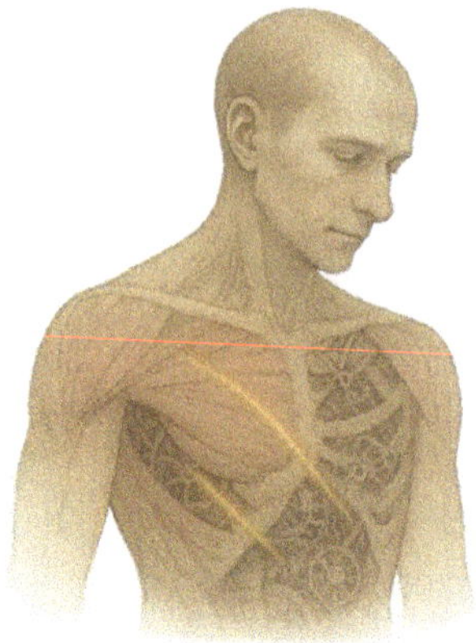

Rafael is forty-three, living with Becker muscular dystrophy. The disease has been wearing away his strength since adolescence, quietly but without pause. By now he moves with the soft hum of an electric wheelchair, his arms thin but still precise. When he enters the office, he apologizes for taking time to park. His tone is even, practiced. He says, *"The pain's back again. Mostly at night. It's not terrible, just endless."*

Leaves: muscle pain and cramps; shallow, broken sleep; exhaustion far beyond physical exertion; panic when breathing tightens at night; visible wasting and increasing dependence on others.

As he speaks, I feel the air in the room grow dense. My own body responds, a slight tightening in the chest, a pull between empathy and fatigue. It is not his defense that tires me; he does not fight or idealize, and he does not pull me into rescue. The exhaustion comes from something quieter: the weight of his realism. There is nothing to interpret away, no hope to sell. He tells his story without drama. As a child, he was "the careful one." He fell often, but smiled after each fall. The diagnosis came at twelve. By twenty, he had learned to disguise weakness with competence. The shift to the wheelchair in his thirties was planned like a project, efficient, clean, mourned in silence. *"You get used to losing things,"* he says, *"you just don't get faster at it."*

Trunk:
Control is both structure and strain. He tracks every muscle, every cramp. He reads new research and corrects his physiotherapist kindly but firmly. When aides in the residential home offer help too soon, he declines with grace. *"Let me try first."* His independence is fierce, but it carries fatigue as its shadow. After sessions I used to feel drained, not frustrated, just hollow. It was a fatigue that came from sitting near something unfixable. Over time, that changed. I learned to stop leaning forward, to let the space breathe. I no longer left the room heavy. Presence itself became lighter when I stopped fighting what could not move.

Roots and soil:
There is no family pathology beyond the gene. The soil is social: the institution's rhythm, the polite monotony of care, peers fading beside him, caregivers rotating through shifts. It is a world that tests dignity daily.

Therapy moved between thought and body. Sometimes we analyzed, sometimes we simply sat through the pain wave. I shifted methods depending on the day: regulation, supportive conversation, small body cues. He followed without complaint, curious about every new approach. Gradually, his sleep improved. The night panic receded. Pain stayed, but lost its accusation. He said, *"It's still there, but it doesn't feel like it's winning."* I noticed I could sit with him longer without the inner drag. My breathing matched his, slower and steadier. He once said, *"You look less tired lately. Maybe you got used to me."* I smiled. *"Maybe I stopped trying to outpace you."* We both laughed. The room felt lighter, not healed, but real. The work had done what medicine rarely can: eased the fight, not by curing, but by staying long enough for both of us to stop resisting the limits.

His tree of symptoms was built long ago. What mattered now was keeping it alive to change with the seasons. But what if what appears broken is simply built differently? Let's look at Paula's case.

Case: The Railway Direction

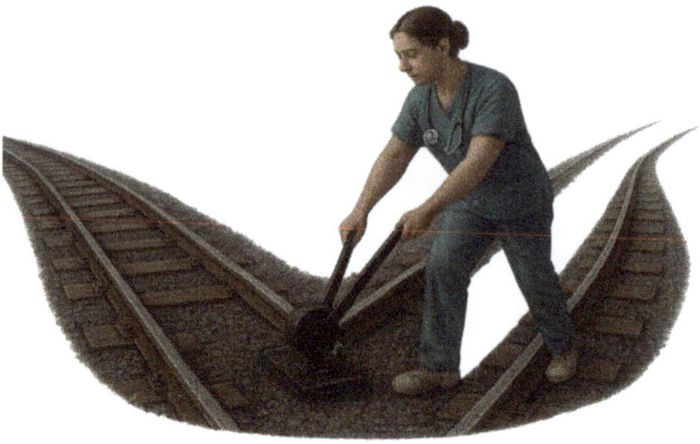

Paula is forty-two when she comes with widespread pain. She describes burning in her shoulders, aching in her legs, and stiffness in the mornings. There are more leaves as well: fatigue, poor concentration, and non-restorative sleep. Her rheumatologic, neurologic, and imaging studies reveal no abnormalities. The diagnosis fits fibromyalgia syndrome. We start with psychoeducation, stress reduction, and body-oriented therapy.

Leaves: widespread pain, fatigue, poor concentration, non-restorative sleep.

At first there is mild improvement. Her sleep deepens, her fatigue lightens, but the pain remains. When the leaves do not fall, you look deeper into the tree. Over months, a different pattern begins to show. Paula calls herself "rigid." She eats the same breakfast every day, avoids changes in routine, and becomes tense when plans shift. At work she is known as "smart but difficult": precise, focused, but easily overwhelmed in group settings. At first I think of personality style: perfectionism, anxious-avoidant traits. Yet the pieces do not fit the usual map. The pattern feels older than defense, as if woven into her way of perceiving.

Trunk: lifelong rigidity, narrow interests, social difficulty, sensory sensitivity, early stress from being misunderstood.

From early childhood, she was described as solitary and precise. Noise and touch overwhelmed her. Friendship was effortful. These are not compensations but development itself. The picture points toward a neurodevelopmental difference, not a trauma adaptation. I refer her to a neuropsychologist for formal assessment, since I do not have full diagnostic training in autism myself. While waiting for the report, I notice my own reactions. I catch myself softening my tone, simplifying phrases, pausing longer. Sessions become structured almost by instinct. The rhythm feels calmer, yet I sense my own tension to "get it right." Working with her precision triggers my own. I leave the room alert and slightly fatigued, as though I have been performing a delicate instrument piece.

Roots: neurodevelopmental vulnerability consistent with autism spectrum.

When the report arrives, the diagnosis is confirmed: ASD (Autism Spectrum Disorder), in her case, corresponding to what was formerly called Asperger's. She receives the news with surprising calm. *"I always suspected something,"* she says. *"Now it makes sense."* I feel a quiet relief, mixed with humility; relief that her story fits at last, humility that I had missed it for months. Paula grew up with parents who valued order and silence. They did not grasp her sensitivities. Their love was steady but structured; affection was practical, not emotional. She learned competence early but never safety in confusion.

Soil: limited parental understanding, chronic family stress, probable intergenerational repetition of similar traits unrecognized.

Therapy changes course. We stop pushing for emotional catharsis and focus on reducing sensory load, managing social strain, and designing routines that fit her rather than fight her. She joins an autism support group and experiments with brief relaxation instead of full body scans, which overwhelm her. Her pain does not vanish, but its grip loosens. She begins to describe sleep that feels "real." When she says, *"I am not broken, just wired differently,"* I feel my own shoulders drop. The diagnosis has given us both permission to stop forcing depth where structure was the issue, to work with what is instead of what should be.

This case taught me that not every rigidity or detachment hides trauma. Sometimes it is neurodevelopmental architecture mistaken for defense. My countertransference, fatigue, over-adjustment, the sense of walking on eggshells, mirrored what she feels in the social world. Once I recognized that, my stance relaxed and the sessions breathed. Understanding the root changed everything: the therapy became supportive rather than corrective, structured rather than interpretive.

Once you see that rigidity can be wiring, not defense, therapy shifts from repair to respect. But what if that wiring has been shattered by violence, and the self had to split to survive? Let's look at Karim's case.

Case: Layers of Survival

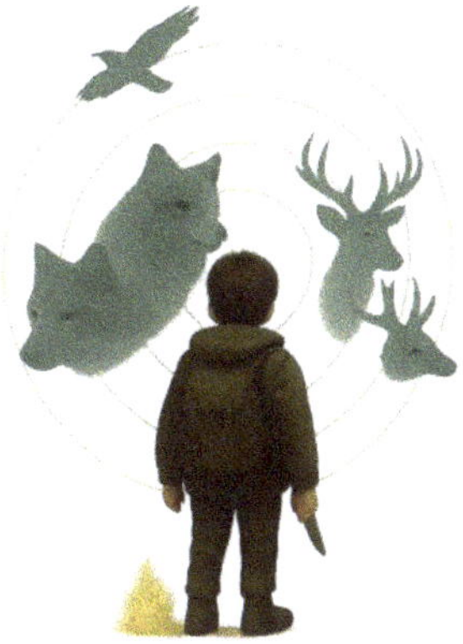

Karim is thirty-six when he comes with chronic dizziness and fatigue. *"It feels like I am not really here,"* he says. *"Like the ground is moving."* Other leaves appear as well: headaches, skin itching, and muscle aches.

Leaves: dizziness, fatigue, headaches, skin itching, muscle pain.

He has lived inside psychiatry for most of his life, moving in and out of wards and programs since his teens. Each stop brought a new label: depression, anxiety, somatization, sometimes suspected psychosis. Medications were started, stopped, and switched. Nothing held. Psychiatry became the only language anyone used for his suffering. I listen closely and more clues surface: episodes of lost time, feeling detached from his body, memory gaps. This points to dissociation, not only anxiety. We look down the tree. Over time, his development comes into focus. Childhood carried neglect, violence, and emotional chaos. Dissociation began as survival, a way to leave the body when reality became unbearable. In adulthood, a violent situation added more trauma. Out of that storm, strategies hardened: sudden anger, unstable relationships, and defensive narcissism. They kept him alive then; now they keep the crisis cycle turning.

Trunk: childhood neglect and violence, dissociation, unstable relationships, defensive narcissism.

Still, something is missing. The roots show what was always there but never named: lifelong ADHD. Restlessness, forgetfulness, and impulsive choices have followed him since childhood, but no one tested him. A fast, easily flooded system kept the stress response humming and kept chaos close.

Roots: ADHD; impulsivity; restlessness.

And the soil reminds us that trauma did not start with him. His mother lived through abuse from his grandfather. Stress travels through families in stories and in chemistry.

Soil: maternal abuse, epigenetic vulnerability, transgenerational trauma.

Only now does the whole tree make sense. We do not fragment care this time. One map, one team, step by step. With psychiatry, social work, and medical colleagues, we build a net: stable housing, financial support, and reliable follow-up. For the first time he says, *"I do not have to fight alone."* Safety becomes the floor. Then, proper testing confirms ADHD. Medication and structure reduce chaos and cut unnecessary emergency visits. Once his life became more stable, he began trauma-focused therapy with a psychotherapist trained in EMDR. EMDR, or Eye Movement Desensitization and Reprocessing, helps the brain process traumatic memories that were previously stuck or fragmented. Along with grounding techniques and strategies to calm an overactive stress system, this work helped Karim feel more present and less drained.

After the trauma treatment, what remained was a clearer underlying pattern: a dissociative disorder as defined in ICD-11, such as Dissociative Identity Disorder or Partial DID. This condition, previously known as multiple personality disorder, involves distinct states of consciousness that can take turns influencing behavior, emotion, or perception. In therapy, we often saw different sides of him functioning, each with its own tone, memory, and way of coping. To make sense of these shifts, we used the concept of "modes" from schema therapy, framing them not as separate selves but as parts of one system that had learned to divide experience in order to survive. This is not "just trauma." It is a long-term structure: the mind compartmentalizing experience to survive. Recognizing it clarifies the task. Treatment shifts toward long-horizon personality work and building stable relationships.

Dizziness and fatigue improve. Hospitalizations fall. He builds routines, works part-time, and, most importantly, starts to trust treatment. This process unfolded over several years, and while he never fully recovered, his relationship with psychiatry changed. It was no longer his whole world, but a steady source of support he could rely on when needed.

Seeing the whole tree matters, and so does an all-in-one approach. Not endless admissions and shifting labels, but one coherent map with coordinated care. In ICD-11, dissociative disorders, including DID and Partial DID, sit in direct relation to severe trauma: a protective split that later traps the adult in crisis loops. Narcissistic defenses can be read the same way, as armor over old wounds, useful once and costly now. Possible psychotic symptoms require careful differentiation. Some are primary psychotic disorders. Others are trauma-related states where perception floods and distance from reality becomes a temporary refuge. The point is not to collapse categories, but to map the whole system before you treat. If you treat one piece, the patient returns. If you integrate the lot and provide steady, trustworthy care, real progress becomes possible, even after a lifetime of fragmented help. Not every health system can offer this level of care to one person, but if you think about it, the many years of fragmented therapy likely cost the system even more in the end.

When survival no longer demands division, the work turns toward integration and trust. But what if intelligence covers a system that can't stop crying out? Let's look at Anastasia's case.

Case: Hidden Behind Brilliance

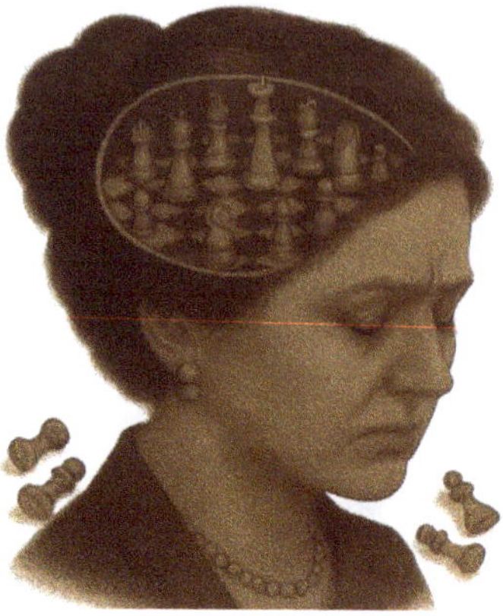

Anastasia is fifty when she comes to us. Her main complaints are chronic fatigue, migraines, diffuse body pain, and insomnia; the familiar leaves of psychosomatic medicine. Her medical file is thick. Over the years she has seen countless specialists, always with the same result: "tests normal." Nothing explains the persistence of her suffering. When she speaks, her brilliance strikes first. Articulate, exact, fast. Sentences build arguments rather than connection. It feels more like being lectured to than confided in. Many doctors before us felt dismissed or corrected by her, and the therapeutic alliance often collapsed before it began.

Leaves: fatigue, migraines, diffuse body pain, insomnia.

Still, the leaves alone do not tell the story. We look deeper. Anastasia was adopted as a baby. Her adoptive parents were kind but overwhelmed, and she grew up feeling like a guest in her own home. At school she stood out, admired for intelligence, excluded for difference. Other children mocked her; teachers praised her but failed to understand her. She learned early that her mind was her safest place. Thinking became armor.

Trunk: childhood stress, feeling misunderstood, survival through intellect.

Since early childhood, there were subtle signs of ADHD (forgetfulness, restlessness, impulsivity) and clear traits on the autism spectrum (sensory sensitivity, narrow focus, rigid routines). Her high IQ masked them all. She compensated through intellect, passing as "high-functioning" while her nervous system ran on overdrive her whole life.

Roots: ADHD; autism spectrum traits; high intelligence as compensation.

Little is known about her biological family, though traces suggest a history of trauma and mental illness. Adoption gave her stability but also distance, a safety gained at the cost of belonging.

Soil: unknown biological history, possible intergenerational trauma.

For years, therapy circled without touching the core. She moved from one clinician to another, always "too complex," always "resistant." Her intellectual style kept others at a distance. Beneath the armor lay isolation, fatigue, and pain. Over time, the puzzle aligned. ADHD was confirmed and treated; structure replaced chaos. Autism traits were recognized; sensory overload was addressed. Trauma therapy allowed her to process the neglect and alienation that shaped her early years. Gradually, the picture grew quieter. Moments of detachment, mild dissociative states, became rare. Her defensiveness softened. Relationships that once collapsed under tension began to hold. These patterns had always been there, not as pathology but the way she had held herself together. The real change came when she found community: others who shared her intelligence and neurodivergent wiring. For the first time she said, *"It's not that I was impossible. I just never belonged to the right tribe."* Her pain and fatigue still return under stress, but now she has a map. For Anastasia, belonging itself became therapy, the one she had been waiting for all along.

Anastasia's case shows how intelligence can disguise vulnerability. High IQ can hide ADHD, autism, trauma, and attachment wounds, and mislead clinicians. Such patients can sound like colleagues: fluent, analytical, self-possessed. Yet intellect often doubles as defense. They explain instead of feel, clarify instead of connect. Countertransference here is subtle. At first, I felt intellectually engaged but emotionally flat, drawn into analysis, not presence. Emotion-focused therapy was difficult at the beginning. Her IQ (intelligence quotient) was high, but her EQ (emotional quotient) was underdeveloped. The alliance deepened when I stopped debating and began witnessing. Giftedness does not protect against psychosomatic illness. In fact, it can intensify it. When intellect becomes the only safe refuge, the body carries what the mind refuses to feel. Roughly two percent of the population falls into the gifted range. You have met these patients before; articulate, demanding, hard to argue with reasoning. When symptoms do not fit and progress feels strangely intellectual, consider the intelligence defense. Beneath it, a nervous system is crying out to be seen, long past the point of words.

After all the theories and treatments, what remains is a human being, like we all are, carrying their stories and scars, searching quietly for the meaning of life.

Your Perspective, Your Practice

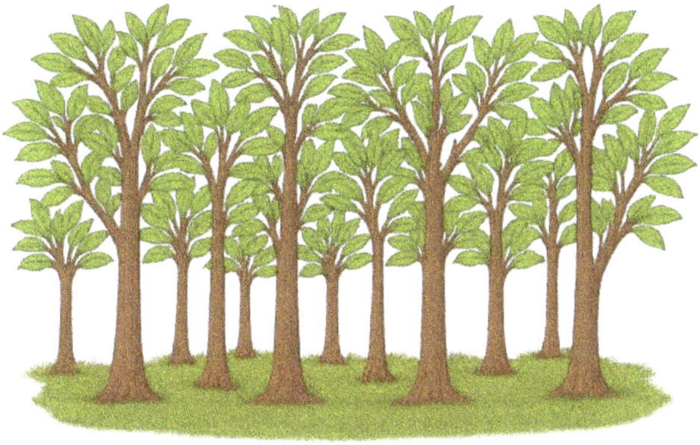

We are all part of the same forest. Each patient is like a tree, their life a world of struggle, resilience, and quiet growth. Some trees bend under storms, some crack, some stretch in directions we cannot foresee. When a patient doesn't get better, the key question is not *"What is wrong with the patient?"* but *"Where in the tree did I stop looking?"* Sometimes the soil is dry. Sometimes the roots are tangled. Sometimes we forget to step back and see the whole shape again. Even if there is nothing more to repair, the act of asking sharpens your eye. That curiosity, calm and steady, is what makes a five-star clinician.

But this does not mean you should turn that precision against yourself. Obsessing over every patient, carrying their stories home, trying to fix everything, is not mastery, it is exhaustion. You are part of the same forest. The same laws apply. When you leave work, leave the other trees to rest. Live your own life with the same rhythm you offer others. Because balance is part of competence. Detailed thinking at work, peace in private life. Settle what needs settling. Build routines that hold you steady. Regulate your own life. The clearer your own soil becomes, the clearer your clinical eye will grow.

That is how we truly give the best care: not by working more, but by listening to our own needs, nurturing our own stability, and bringing our full presence to each patient and each moment.

Final Note

At first, I drew the Tree simply to make sense of complexity. Patients came with overlapping symptoms, multiple diagnoses, and stories that refused simple categories. Lists and checkboxes could not hold them, but a tree could. Suddenly, everything belonged to one living structure. Patients saw their illness not as fragments, but as form.

As my work deepened with Schema Therapy and ISTDP, the image evolved. Schema Therapy gave the Tree its voices, the modes that speak in the language of lived experience. ISTDP revealed its fire, the movement of feeling, defense, and anxiety shaping symptoms in real time. At first, I used these models separately. Over years, they began to merge. When I showed how modes bend the triangle or how the branches of history sustain the leaves of the present, patients understood. Their suffering became traceable, even changeable. Eventually, I realized I was no longer switching between theories. I was watching one movement expressed through different forms. Sometimes I spoke of the triangle, sometimes the tree, sometimes the inner figures that travel between them. The image held everything: dynamic, symbolic, alive.

It was my patients who convinced me to share it. The Tree of Symptoms helped them first, then began to help colleagues. It offered a language that crossed disciplines, joining biology, psychology, and relationship into one coherent frame.

I invite you to test these perspectives in your own practice. Use simple language. Let patients find themselves in it. Notice how they respond, whether with resistance, relief, or new understanding. And if what you observe differs from what I have written, even better. Write it down. Refine it. Let it grow into your own version.

This is not a method to follow.
It is a map to redraw.
Your eyes. Your patients. Your practice.

References and Suggested Reading

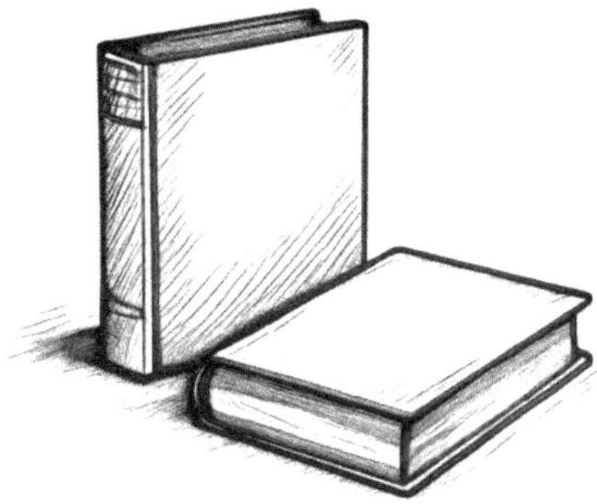

Abbass, A. (2015). *Reaching Through Resistance: Advanced Psychotherapy Techniques.* Seven Leaves Press.

Abbass, A. (2018). *Hidden from View: Clinician's Guide to Psychophysiologic Disorders.* Seven Leaves Press.

American Psychiatric Association (2022). *Diagnostic and Statistical Manual of Mental Disorders (5th ed., text rev.).* American Psychiatric Publishing.

Beck, J. S. (2011). *Cognitive Behavior Therapy: Basics and Beyond (2nd ed.).* Guilford Press.

Blackburn, E. H., & Epel, E. S. (2017). *The Telomere Effect: A Revolutionary Approach to Living Younger, Healthier, Longer.* Grand Central Publishing.

Davanloo, H. (1990). *Unlocking the Unconscious: Selected Papers of Habib Davanloo, MD.* John Wiley & Sons.

Egle, U. T., Heim, C., Strauß, B., & von Känel, R. (Eds.) (2024). *Psychosomatik: Neurobiologisch fundiert und evidenzbasiert (2nd ed.).* Kohlhammer.

Egloff, N., Sütterlin, S., & von Känel, R. (2012). *The clothes peg as a simple screening instrument for central sensitization syndromes.* Psychosomatics, 53(5), 451–454.

Fonagy, P., Gergely, G., Jurist, E. L., & Target, M. (2002). *Affect Regulation, Mentalization, and the Development of the Self.* Other Press.

Frederickson, J. (2013). *Co-Creating Change: Effective Dynamic Therapy Techniques.* Seven Leaves Press.

Frederickson, J. (2024). *Clinical Thinking in Psychotherapy: What It Is, How It Works, and Why and How to Teach It.* Routledge.

Lanius, R. A., Vermetten, E., & Pain, C. (Eds.). (2010). *The Impact of Early Life Trauma on Health and Disease: The Hidden Epidemic.* Cambridge University Press.

Lane, R. D., & Nadel, L. (Eds.). (2000). *Cognitive Neuroscience of Emotion.* Oxford University Press.

McEwen, B. S. (2007). *Physiology and neurobiology of stress and adaptation: Central role of the brain.* Physiological Reviews, 87(3), 873–904.

Meaney, M. J., & Szyf, M. (Eds.). (2015). *Epigenetics and Neuroendocrinology.* Springer.

Moseley, L., & Butler, D. (2015). *Explain Pain (2nd ed.).* Noigroup Publications.

Neisser, U., Boodoo, G., Bouchard, T. J., Boykin, A. W., Brody, N., Ceci, S. J., Halpern, D. F., Loehlin, J. C., Perloff, R., Sternberg, R. J., & Urbina, S. (1996). *Intelligence: Knowns and unknowns.* American Psychologist, 51(2), 77–101.

Porges, S. W. (2011). *The Polyvagal Theory: Neurophysiological Foundations of Emotions, Attachment, Communication, and Self-Regulation.* W. W. Norton.

Sapolsky, R. M. (2004). *Why Zebras Don't Get Ulcers (3rd ed.).* Holt.

van der Kolk, B. A. (2014). *The Body Keeps the Score: Brain, Mind, and Body in the Healing of Trauma.* Viking.

World Health Organization. (2022). *International Classification of Diseases for Mortality and Morbidity Statistics (11th Revision).*

Young, J. E., Klosko, J. S., & Weishaar, M. E. (2003). *Schema Therapy: A Practitioner's Guide.* Guilford Press.

About the Author

Emil Šabanović, MD, is a specialist in psychiatry, psychotherapy, psychosomatic and psychosocial medicine.
He lives and works in Switzerland, where he also teaches and writes about mind–body integration.

www.sabanovic.online

www.ingramcontent.com/pod-product-compliance
Lightning Source LLC
Chambersburg PA
CBHW041303210926
51850CB00001B/3
9783033119147